Diabetes
& the Metabolic Syndrome

D, APD)

To mum & dad who gave so much...

Acknowledgements

I gratefully acknowledge the help and support of the following team members:

Linda Turner RN (Registered Nurse), CDE (Credentialed Diabetes Educator), Previous Manager of the Diabetes Centre, Prince of Wales Hospital (POWH) Randwick NSW 2031, Australia. Former president of the Australian Diabetes Educators Association (ADEA) NSW.

Professor Stephen Colagiuri MBBS, FRACP. Endocrinologist. Professor of Metabolic Health, Sydney University. Previous director of the Diabetes Centre, The Prince of Wales Hospital, Randwick NSW 2031, Australia. Co-author of 'The Glucose Revolution' and 'The GI Factor' and 'The New Glucose Revolution'.

Professor Bernard Tuch FRACP, PhD. Endocrinologist. Professor Department of Endocrinology, Diabetes and Metabolism, The Prince of Wales Hospital, Randwick NSW 2031, Australia.

Dr Vernon Naidu MBBS, FRACP. Endocrinologist, Diabetes Centre, POWH.

Dr Kenneth Chen MBBS, FRACP. Endocrinologist, Diabetes Centre, POWH.

Kirsty Boltong RN, CDE, Present Manager of the Diabetes Centre, POWH.

Michelle Redmond RN, CDE, CNS (Clinical Nurse Specialist), Diabetes Centre, POWH.

Charmaine DeBlieck RN, CDE, CNC (Clinical Nurse Consultant), Diabetes Centre, POWH.

Julie Cadman B.Med.Sc. Research assistant.

Monique Etkind. Dietitian.

Marianne Byrne. Dietitian.

Jayne McGreal. Podiatrist, Diabetes Centre, POWH.

Cherie Campbell RN, CDE, Diabetes Centre, POWH.

Chris Tzar. Exercise physiologist. Director, The Lifestyle Clinic, Faculty of Medicine, University of NSW, Sydney, NSW Australia.

Marcus Cremonese. Head graphic designer and his team of photographers, graphic artists at the Medical Illustrations Unit at the University of New South Wales, Faculty of Medicine and Teaching Hospitals for their patience, cooperation and professional work in developing the 'Healthy Food Pyramid', its tiers, the 'Plate Model' and Glycemic Index (GI) figures.

Margaret Gee. Author and literary agent—for her guidance, support and constant encouragement.

Nadine Davidoff. Freelance editor who has worked as a senior editor for Random House Australia for her encouragement and editorial feedback.

Julie Middleton and dietitians at Diabetes Australia Western Australia for the idea of using photographs to visually illustrate fat and sugar in food.

My son **Dimitri** and daughter **Sara** for their help in designing the title page.

My beautiful wife **Nayla** for her simple recipes, her love and never-ending support and encouragement.

My patients for their constant source of inspiration.

Contents

Figures & Illustrations

34. The sugar (white) and fat (yellow) in Tim Tam™ biscuits
35. The high content of oil in nuts
36. The high caloric content of nuts
37. The high content of oil in avocados
38. The high caloric content of avocados
39. The pure fat content of oil
40. The high caloric density of oil

List of Tables

Foreword

We are confronted on a daily basis by the alarming increase in obesity, heart disease and diabetes. Today's global society seems to have lost touch with its natural body rhythms.

By contrasting today's activity and nutritional problems against nature's own template for our health, as hunter/gatherers, Dr Malouf has put into a readable and informative text an invaluable tool that will help us to get back to basics, and to eat nature's foods that are designed for the health of our body.

For those with and at risk of diabetes and it's associated Metabolic Syndrome risk factors (obesity, high blood sugars, high blood pressure and abnormal blood fats), Dr Malouf has applied the hunter/gatherer approach to each aspect of these serious issues affecting health outcomes and has provided a commonsense, practical and applicable solution.

For health care professionals teaching nutritional guidelines and also for those exposed to energy-dense food, sedentary lifestyles and complicated and confusing dietary advice, this book simply makes sense.

Linda Turner CDE (Credentialed Diabetes Educator)
Former Manager Diabetes Centre
Prince of Wales Hospital (POWH)
Randwick NSW 2031
AUSTRALIA

Former President of Australian Diabetes Educators Association (ADEA), NSW.

Testimonials

M Byrne (Dietitian—BSc Nutrition, Hons, University of Sydney).
This book cuts through much of the confusion surrounding diabetes management by explaining, in a straightforward and easy to understand manner, complex but fundamental concepts. The rationale behind suggested dietary and activity modifications is logically described and then applied through practical and pragmatic advice and guidance, which will prove invaluable to people with diabetes and health professionals alike. The core principle of the hunter/gatherer paradigm on which the book is built provides a strong backbone to return to in understanding the prevention and management of Metabolic Syndrome risk factors in diabetes.

M Fosh (Patient with Type 2 diabetes).
As a person with diabetes, I found the book easy to follow and understand as a no-nonsense approach to healthy living. It's outstanding! An essential read for any person with diabetes. It makes simple what other books make complicated. Healthy lifestyle tips are supplemented with examples from cultures, which don't have the complications that are on the rise in our society. Forget the cabbage and protein diets—this is a lifestyle and it works. It is full of wisdom and practical advice with a light touch. A hunting and gathering I go!

D Janssen (Visiting 4th year medical student from Maastricht, the Netherlands).
This book by Dr Malouf is clear and inviting to read. It is explained in an easy and understandable way. As a medical student, I believe that it will be of great use in understanding the basics of lifestyle issues in diabetes management for both doctors and patients alike.

R Crawford (Patient with Type 2 diabetes).
As a person who has recently been diagnosed with Type 2 diabetes, I found your book very interesting and informative. It's easy to read and answered all of my questions about diabetes. The concept of the hunter/gatherer, together with the new pictorial Food Pyramid allowed me to reassess my diet and make the necessary adjustments to

my meal planning. The importance of exercise is clearly explained and very encouraging. I have previously found exercise quite difficult, as I have arthritis in most joints. However, I felt motivated after reading your book and I went and purchased a kick board and goggles and plan to have a daily swim (keeping my fingers crossed that I don't sink!). I am sure this lifestyle book will be a valuable reference for those who are living with diabetes, family members who care for them and allied health practitioners.

K Baker (Dietitian—Masters in Nutrition and Dietetics, University of Sydney).
This book is a very useful resource for any person interested in preventing or managing diabetes and its associated Metabolic Syndrome risk factors—obesity, lipids and blood pressure. It discusses key concepts in a comprehensive yet easy to understand manner, and provides realistic and achievable solutions for a healthier lifestyle. Comparison of the typical modern day diet and lifestyle with that of our hunter/gatherer ancestors provides a fascinating insight into some of the factors contributing to these current diet/lifestyle-related diseases.

C Campbell (RN, CDE).
Diabetes has reached epidemic proportions in Western societies, with many misconceptions surrounding the management of it and its Metabolic Syndrome risk factors. This book is an excellent resource as it explains in an easy to understand manner, to the health professional or lay person, how important the Metabolic Syndrome is in managing diabetes. The hunter/gatherer is an excellent concept, which demonstrates how lifestyle factors of the 20th and 21st centuries have impacted so greatly on our bodies, causing chronic diseases such as diabetes. This book utilises evidence-based practice literature on how to effectively implement important lifestyle changes. It contains great information which is practical and achievable for anyone who wishes to learn how to self manage the life-long challenges they will need to address and sustain to prevent, delay or control diabetes.

About the Author

Dr Nasseem Michael Malouf (PhD, MSc, BSc) is a team member of the Diabetes Centre, Department of Endocrinology, Diabetes and Metabolism at The Prince of Wales Hospital, Randwick, New South Wales, Sydney, Australia. He is also an Accredited Practising Dietitian (APD) and an Accredited Nutritionist (AN) and has been working in diabetes education privately and publicly for 25 years. He first worked at the Diabetes Education Center, Royal North Shore Hospital, St Leonards, Sydney, Australia, until 1991. In 1991, he joined The Prince of Wales Hospital diabetes team. He has spent most of his working life in education of patients and health professionals (dietitians, podiatrists, medical doctors, nurse educators) working or training in the area of diabetes management. He is actively involved with the Human Nutrition Unit at The University of Sydney in training dietitians as part of their practical placements. He has developed several dietary resources used in diabetes education now Australia wide.

He has been a member of the Board of Directors of Diabetes Australia, NSW, and is presently a member of the Dietitians Association of Australia and the NSW Diabetes, Obesity and Cardiology Special Interest Groups. He has recently worked as a research officer reviewing the evidence that culminated in the Diabetes Australia, NHMRC Guidelines for the Management of Lipids (blood fats) in Type 2 diabetes.

He is a regular guest speaker on SBS Radio, increasing awareness of lifestyle issues in public health. He was a presenter in the past on a 13-part lifestyle program called '*Second Opinion*' on SBS Television. He is also a presenter on a 13-part healthy cooking series called '*To Good Health*' which has screened in many countries overseas.

He is a firm believer in the old cliché 'you are what you eat' and that diet, together with regular activity, is essential in the treatment of today's chronic degenerative diseases but more importantly in their prevention. He walks regularly, rides bikes and swims for aerobic fitness and attends a gym regularly for strength and flexibility training.

He is a NSW state champion in American skeet—a discipline of clay target shooting. He also enjoys other clay target disciplines like trap, field and game and five stand. He has co-directed a documentary on American skeet here in Australia called '*Over & Down Under*'.

He is a keen photographer of landscapes, portraits and—believe it or not—food. He lives with his wife Nayla and kids—Sara and Dimitri—in Sydney.

Introduction

Humans have been hunter/gatherers for 98 per cent of their time on earth and have evolved over at least 2.6 million years to adapt to lack of food and even famine in order to survive in the wild. However, this is quite unsuited to our modern lifestyle of affluence and abundance. We today have diverged from Nature's Laws; a sedentary lifestyle and a highly refined and processed diet. Unfortunately, we are paying a high price for this with modern diseases like Type 2 diabetes, obesity and heart disease. In contrast to what we see in developing nations and Western countries, these diseases are rarely seen in traditional societies and even more rarely in present hunter-gatherer societies. [1]

Compare these two scenarios. A tribesman's existence evolves around hunting and gathering for food just to survive. He spends much of his day walking and running anything from 8 to 16 kilometres to find enough food for the family—and that is just for the next meal. His food is largely natural, eaten in its unprocessed unrefined form. He gathers seeds, nuts and berries. He digs for tubers but mostly hunts for wild lean game. He cooks it fresh, no fats, preservatives or additives to be seen—as Nature provided it. His caloric intake is limited as he has to share his food with many in the tribe. He drinks fresh water to quench his thirst, and even that he had to fetch from the nearby stream. He has the occasional *acute* stress episode as he experiences the *fight or flight* response to dangers he occasionally encounters along the way. He has to do this every day, rain, hail or sunshine, otherwise he and his family would starve. He has no choice. He may be malnourished but you can understand why he is lean and mean and does not suffer from the diseases of affluence we suffer from today such as obesity, diabetes and heart disease.

In contrast, our modern day middle-aged, single stockbroker rises early in the morning to face another day with no time to make breakfast. Instead he drives his Merc to the nearest Arches and purchases a 600 Calorie (2510 kilojoules) breakfast of food his hunter/gatherer counterpart would not even recognise, let alone eat. He hasn't spent a calorie yet. He copes with the stress of driving to work by ingesting his Sausage McMuffin and hash browns and helping it down with an artificially coloured strawberry shake loaded with sugar. He then sits at his desk for 10 hours staring at a computer screen watching the fluctuating stock market. He is *chronically* stressed. He can't wait for the biscuit trolley to come around; he sips his Coke all day and takes regular breaks to puff on cancer sticks. He returns home having to go through all that driving again.

It's too late for cooking so he picks up a Chinese takeaway on the way, and who knows how that was cooked. He puts his feet up and unwinds with a few ales. He has walked no more than 3000 steps (the equivalent of 2 kilometres) all day. Any excuse for not doing any exercise will do—a cloud over the next continent is a good enough excuse not to go out for a walk. He retires only to wake up the next morning to go through the same routine again. No wonder he, unlike our hunter/gatherer tribesman, has the early signs of sugar problems or pre-diabetes, high blood fats, high blood pressure and central (abdominal) obesity—all the risk factors of the Metabolic Syndrome.

Humans largely evolved during the Palaeolithic hunter/gatherer period that stretched from 2.6 million years to 40,000 years ago. They emerged from this period with the appearance of truly modern human beings, *Homo sapiens sapiens*. Evidence has shown that our genes have not changed significantly since this time [2] but our diet and activity levels have progressively diverged from that of our ancient ancestors with technological, social, environmental and economic changes. Significant changes occurred with the Agricultural Revolution, 10,000 years ago, and more so with the first Industrial Revolution 250 years ago. The most dramatic changes though have occurred in the past 100 years.

Diabetes is only one of the chronic degenerative diseases increasing at an alarming rate as a result of these lifestyle changes (see Chapter 1). There are two main types of diabetes—Type 1 and Type 2 and a temporary form, gestational diabetes.

Type 1 diabetes, the less common form that affects 10 to 15 per cent of all cases, is an auto-immune disease. That simply means that the cells in the pancreas that produce insulin are destroyed by the body's own immune system. Its onset is sudden and dramatic and occurs mainly in the young and for that reason is commonly known as Juvenile Onset Diabetes. It is also known as Insulin Dependant Diabetes Mellitus (IDDM) because daily insulin injections are required for survival.

Type 2 diabetes is the more common form of the disease affecting 85 to 90 per cent of all people with diabetes. Unlike Type 1, Type 2 diabetes is a lifestyle disease. It occurs largely in adults with a family history. That is why, until recently, it has been referred to as Adult Onset Diabetes. However, no longer is it referred to as such since recently it is increasingly being found in obese, inactive young adults and even adolescents. [3, 4, 5] Alarmingly, these adolescents have been found to have significantly higher rates of diabetes complications compared to their peers with Type 1 despite a much shorter duration of the disease. [6]

> Unlike Type 1 diabetes, Type 2 diabetes is a lifestyle disease that is theoretically preventable

> » **Gestational diabetes** is a temporary form of the disease that occurs during pregnancy due to hormonal changes that prevent the insulin that is normally produced by the body from doing its job. Most women restore normal insulin function and normal blood sugar levels after delivery. However, if they don't implement some serious lifestyle changes, more than 50 per cent go on to develop Type 2 diabetes within 10 years.

Type 2 diabetes, is caused by a gradual reduction in the amount of insulin the pancreas produces in response to meals and by the insulin resistance that occurs when the normal amount of insulin secreted by the pancreas is unable to perform its job of transferring sugars from the blood stream into muscle and fat cells. Insulin resistance forces the pancreas to produce even higher than normal levels of insulin—a condition called hyperinsulinemia.[7] When insulin levels are consistently elevated, a long list of complications can follow. That is why Type 2 diabetes is often associated with an abnormal metabolic state that is referred to today as the '*Metabolic Syndrome*' also known as '*Syndrome X*' or the '*Insulin Resistance Syndrome*'. This includes a cluster of other abnormalities besides high blood sugars including, among others, abnormal blood fats, high blood pressure and central obesity that is found around the waistline and often referred to as abdominal or visceral (see Chapter 4). This is now thought to be driving the unusually high rate of cardiovascular disease in the diabetes population.

No one knows for sure what causes insulin resistance. Some scientists think it may be a defect in specific genes. What we do know however is that insulin resistance is aggravated by certain lifestyle factors common to Western industrialised and developing nations today—physical inactivity and central obesity being major factors (see Figure 1). Unfortunately, nowadays we are treating the symptoms of Type 2 diabetes, not the cause. What we have to address are the lifestyle issues in order to turn the tide on diabetes and its cardiovascular complications.

Figure 1. The effects of insulin resistance on the Metabolic Syndrome and Diabetes

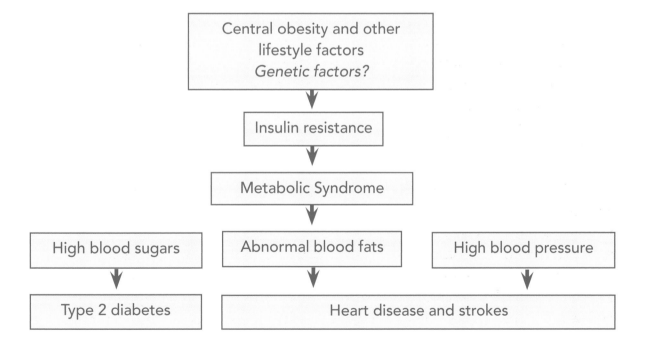

Do you know which lifestyle factors are important in preventing or treating insulin resistance, Type 2 diabetes and the Metabolic Syndrome? Do you have difficulty understanding the dietary factors? Well, join the millions of others today who are constantly being bombarded with information that is not only difficult to understand, but in many cases conflicting. It's a jungle out there and you—like most others—could be lost in this maze of information. Dietary terms that mean nothing to most of us are being used. Terms like energy intake, energy balance, proteins, carbohydrates, monosaccharides, disaccharides, polysaccharides, starches, refined carbohydrates, complex carbohydrates, Glycemic Index (GI), high GI, low GI, Glycemic Load (GL), high GL, low GL, soluble fibre, polyunsaturated fats, monounsaturated fats, saturated fats, omega 3 fats, trans fats, high-protein diets and low-fat diets. Labels are added to food products that most of us have difficulty pronouncing let alone interpreting.

As a health professional working in this field for 25 years, I see how nutrition is made out to be complex and intriguing. It is not surprising to hear of a different diet everyday. One of the most challenging tasks I have experienced in my career is to find a simple way to explain dietary principles that cuts through all the unnecessarily detailed and often conflicting information.

Today we have a much clearer picture of the ideal lifestyle for humans. It is apparent to me that Nature's Laws can explain today's recommended lifestyle principles in an easy way that you can relate to, can learn from and even teach.

I have been using this 'hunter/gatherer' or 'back to basics' concept to explain diet and lifestyle principles for more than 20 years. I have used this in programs for thousands of people with pre-diabetes (early stages of the disease), diabetes and health professionals such as nurses, medical doctors, podiatrists, exercise physiologists, psychologists and dietitians who work in the area of diabetes management. It has proven to be easy, entertaining and most of all effective in getting the message across. I hope you find it that way too.

In Part 1 of this book, I will discuss the modern epidemic of diabetes. I will highlight the importance of addressing Metabolic Syndrome risk factors other than blood sugars (blood pressure, blood fats, central or abdominal obesity) in order to prevent serious complications and touch on the importance of early prevention and what those at risk need to do to turn back the clock. By understanding these fundamental principles you will appreciate the need to make the necessary lifestyle changes explained in Part 2.

In Part 2, I will go 'back to basics' and look at the practical dietary and lifestyle changes needed to realign our modern lifestyle with our ancient genes. This will not only help delay insulin resistance, diabetes and its Metabolic Syndrome risk factors, but hopefully prevent it in the first place.

The reader is advised to consult the Glossary for any necessary explanation or definition of terms that they do not understand.

PART 1

Diabetes and
the Metabolic Syndrome

1: Diabetes—
The modern epidemic

Diabetes (Type 2), along with other modern lifestyle diseases such as coronary heart disease, stroke and some cancers is at epidemic level in the West. These diseases typically affect 50 to 65 per cent of the adult population yet they are rare or non-existent in hunter/gatherer societies. They are also rare in non-Westernised people. Even in Westernised countries, these diseases were rare prior to the turn of the 20th century and are mostly lifestyle related and so theoretically preventable.

How common is diabetes worldwide?

Worldwide, it is estimated there are more than 246 million people with diabetes (about 5 per cent of the adult population) in the year 2007 and that this number is escalating at an alarming rate. In the past few decades, the number of people with diabetes has more than doubled globally. If unchecked, it is expected that diabetes will reach epidemic proportions, affecting 380 million people by the year 2025 [8] (see Figure 2).

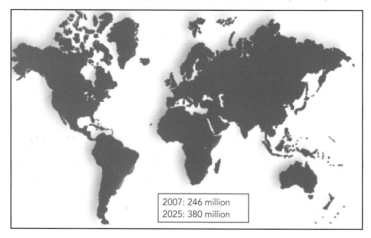

2007: 246 million
2025: 380 million

Figure 2. The prevalence of diabetes worldwide

Approximately 90 per cent of the cases have Type 2 diabetes. For a non-communicable disease, this rate of increase is alarming and represents a serious epidemic with global implications. In December 2006, the United Nations General Assembly unanimously declared diabetes a global public health issue, second only to HIV/AIDS.

Diabetes is increasing at an alarming rate in Westernised countries such as the United States and Australia.

For example, 'approximately one quarter of the Australian population over the age of 25 years are having a problem with glucose tolerance and the potential accompanying health consequences'. The *Australian Diabetes, Obesity and Lifestyle Study* showed that in adults over the age of 25 years, the prevalence was found to be 7.4 per cent in 1999–2000. [9] Furthermore, another 16.4 per cent of the population had Impaired Fasting Glucose (IFG) and/or Impaired Glucose Tolerance (IGT) now known to be pre-diabetic stages. Even in the 25 to 34 year age group, 5.7 per cent already had pre-diabetes. As predicted, those with pre-diabetes were at increased risk of developing full-blown diabetes within the next 5 to10 years if they did not make some serious lifestyle changes. A follow up of this study actually showed just that— those with pre-diabetes were 10 to 20 times more likely to develop diabetes by 2005 compared to those with normal blood sugars.[10] This study also showed that there are now 275 new cases of diabetes every day, making it Australia's fastest growing chronic disease. It is predicted that in the short period between 2006 and 2010 the occurrence of diabetes will grow from 1.4 million to 2 million. This is already a major health crisis and needs to be addressed with urgency as it places a large burden on the health care system. [11]

In the United States, the dramatic increase among adults between 1990 and 2001 is clearly shown in Figure 3.[12, 13, 14] There are now 14.6 million people with diabetes who know they have the disease. Since at least 6.2 million do not know they have it, the actual number with diabetes is more like 21 million, or around 7 per cent of the population. Already, diabetes accounts for 12 per cent of the national health budget in the USA. It is estimated that another 41 million people have pre-diabetes (early stages) and could be on their way to developing the disease unless they make some serious lifestyle changes.

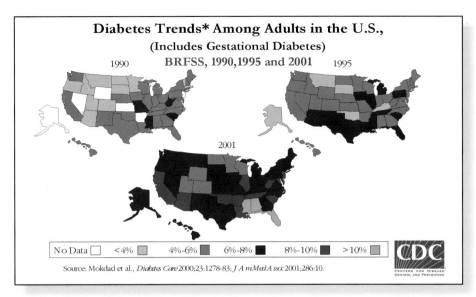

Figure 3.

Diabetes trends among adults in the US from 1990 to 2001.

Reproduced with persmission from CDC.

Why is Type 2 diabetes increasing at such an alarming rate?

The reasons behind the increase worldwide are the consequences of changing lifestyles: increasing urbanisation, unhealthy diets, obesity and sedentary lifestyles.

Urbanisation

Moving from life on the land to the cities is one reason why the number of people with diabetes is rising worldwide. Although urbanisation can be seen as a positive development in many respects, it is the change in eating habits to richer foods containing more energy (calories/kilojoules), saturated fat and sugars, accompanied by less physical activity that leads to a greater chance of getting diabetes. This phenomenon is particularly evident in the rich countries of the Arabian Gulf and highly populated developing nations like India and China where social and economic progress has been dramatic in the past few decades. The peoples of southern Asia, especially Indians, have a very high prevalence of diabetes and the World Health Organization (WHO) estimates that India will soon have the largest number of people with diabetes in the world.

Immigration and adoption of Western lifestyles

We are seeing an increase in diabetes, not only in people who switch from a rural to an urban lifestyle (for example, in India and China), but also in those who immigrate from less affluent countries, for example the Pacific Islands, Asia, Eastern and Southern Europe and the Middle East to the more affluent Western countries such as Australia, the UK, Canada and the United States.

Even within traditional societies around the world there has been an even more dramatic increase in diabetes with the adoption of Western lifestyles. This is obvious in the Pacific Islands (Nauru, Tonga, Fiji etc) and in the Pima Indians of the United States. The Pima Indians have what is known as a 'thrifty gene' which means their metabolism is efficiently geared to laying down fat in preparation for times of famine. Even by age eight, most are already resistant to insulin and on the way to developing diabetes. By old age nearly all have developed Type 2 diabetes. But this plague only struck after the Pima Indians adopted a sedentary lifestyle and ate a typical Western diet high in fat, sugar, refined carbohydrates and low in fibre. Pima Indians who live in the United States have at least a four-fold greater prevalence of diabetes compared with those with similar genetic background living in Mexico.[15] Similarly, Australian urban Aborigines suffer the fourth highest rate of diabetes in the world. In some Aboriginal and Torres Strait Islander communities this incidence of diabetes is as high as 30 per cent, compared to 7.4 per cent in the non-indigenous population.

Overweight and obesity epidemics

The International Obesity Task Force (IOTF) reports that there are 1.7 billion people worldwide at risk of weight-related diseases such as diabetes. In fact, the increase in diabetes parallels the rising rates of obesity and increase in Body Mass Index (BMI) observed over the last decade. The association between Type 2 diabetes and obesity is so strong that together they are often referred to as one disease 'diabesity', the largest epidemic the world is facing in the first two decades of the 21st century'.[17]

However, excess body fat in the central area or abdomen, measured simply by waist circumference, is even more indicative of diabetes and the Metabolic Syndrome than BMI (see Figure 4). There is a direct relationship between increased abdominal weight and insulin resistance, diabetes and cardiovascular risk.[18, 19]

Figure 4. Central or abdominal obesity

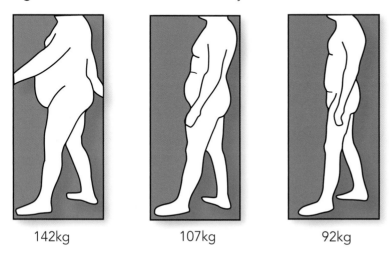

142kg   107kg   92kg

Obesity also complicates the management of diabetes by affecting other Metabolic Syndrome risk factors such as abnormal blood fats and high blood pressure. These increase the risk of the cardiovascular complications of diabetes (heart, stroke, peripheral vascular disease or blocked arteries in the legs).

Obesity in adults is increasing at an alarming rate in most Westernised countries. It has at least doubled between 1991 and 2004 according to figures put out by the Centers for Disease Control (CDC) in Atlanta, USA.

Prior to 1970, about 5 per cent of American children between the ages of 6 and 19 had obesity. By the year 2002, this number had quadrupled to 16 per cent. [20]

In Australia, the figures are no less alarming. As reported in the AusDiab study, obesity has at least doubled in adult males and females in the 20 years to 2000 and almost tripled in children over the same period.[21] This trend is no different in other developed countries. Unless something is done to prevent this epidemic as early as childhood, we can expect diabetes to increase even more in the future.

To prevent the rise and rise of diabetes globally, we need to control the global epidemic of obesity right from the early stages of childhood

Our ageing population

This could partly explain the increase in diabetes in Western countries as the risk of developing Type 2 diabetes increases with age and is much more common in the over 55 age group—an age when most have gained significant weight since their early twenties. Today, however, diabetes is being diagnosed earlier in life largely because of the earlier onset of obesity. In the United States there has been an overall increase in Type 2 diabetes of 32 per cent during the short period of 1990 to 1998, a 40 per cent increase in the 40 to 49-year-old group and an alarming 70 per cent increase in the young 30 to 39-year-old group. As mentioned earlier, we now have a surge in Type 2 diabetes even in overweight children and adolescents.[5]

So the overall increase in Type 2 diabetes is not solely the result of our population living longer.

Can Type 2 diabetes be prevented?

There is strong evidence to suggest that we can prevent diabetes in those who are at risk or seem to be showing early signs of developing the disease (see Table 1).

Recent studies carried out in Finland, the USA, China and India have shown that moderate lifestyle changes—a few less calories, slightly more physical activity and modest weight loss can significantly reduce the chance of developing diabetes in people with a high risk.[22, 23, 24, 25, 26]

In these studies, men and women with pre-diabetes who successfully lost a modest amount of weight (5 to 10 per cent of body weight) using a diet low in fat/high in fibre with regular activity (walking 4 to 5 times per week), managed to reduce their risk of developing Type 2 diabetes by up to 58 per cent. The reduction in the incidence of diabetes was directly associated with lifestyle changes which were far more effective in preventing diabetes than drugs like Biguanides (Metformin™) which are known to improve insulin sensitivity, Acarbose (Glucobay™) a drug that stops the digestion of long chain carbohydrates like starch[27] and Orlistat (commonly known as Xenical™) which prevents the digestion and absorption of fat in the diet. Promising new drugs (Glitazones or Thiazolidinediones, TZDs) have recently been tested[28] but have since been found to have some side effects.

At present we do not have definite proof that Type 2 diabetes can be totally prevented. However, we can 'safely conclude that the current evidence strongly favours the notion that lifestyle changes are the primary means to tackle the epidemic of Type 2 diabetes'.[25]

Small lifestyle changes significantly reduce the risk of developing diabetes

Table 1. High risk categories for developing Type 2 diabetes*

- Anyone over the age of 55 years
- Anyone over the age of 45 years with a weight problem, high blood pressure or a family history of diabetes
- Anyone who has recorded a borderline blood sugar level
- Any woman who has had high blood sugar levels during pregnancy
- Any woman with polycystic ovaries and a weight problem
- Any Aboriginal or Torres Straight Islander over the age of 35 years
- Anyone from the Pacific islands, Indian sub-continent or of Chinese and Middle Eastern cultural background

*Diabetes Australia

2: What is diabetes and how is it diagnosed?

Diabetes, in a nutshell, is a disease where sugars circulating in the blood stream are significantly higher than normal. In order to understand why blood sugars are higher in people with diabetes one must first understand how the body normally handles sugars.

To achieve normal blood sugars your body needs to be able to do two things:

» Release enough insulin from the pancreas at the right time in response to meals. Insulin, secreted by the beta cells in the pancreas, facilitates the entry of sugar (glucose) into fat cells and muscle cells to be used as a source of fuel.

» Insulin secreted into the blood stream must be able to open doors (insulin receptors) on muscle and fat cells to transfer sugar inside them. The more sensitive these cells are to insulin, the easier the process.

What is insulin resistance?

Insulin resistance is the inability of insulin to open these doors to allow the transfer of sugar inside muscle and fat cells. It is aggravated by obesity, particularly central obesity, and lack of activity. Faced with this, in order to maintain normal blood sugar levels, the pancreas compensates by secreting even more insulin, resulting in even higher levels in the bloodstream—a condition called hyperinsulinemia. This in turn causes more doors or receptors on cells to close. As this vicious cycle continues, the pancreas gradually fails to produce enough insulin and glucose builds up in the blood stream, resulting initially in pre-diabetes and eventually in Type 2 diabetes.

Table 2. What happens to blood sugars in diabetes?

Step 1: The small intestine	Carbohydrate foods (cereal products, fruits, starchy vegetables, sugars) are chewed in the mouth and completely broken down or digested largely to a sugar called 'glucose' in the small intestine (see Figure 5) 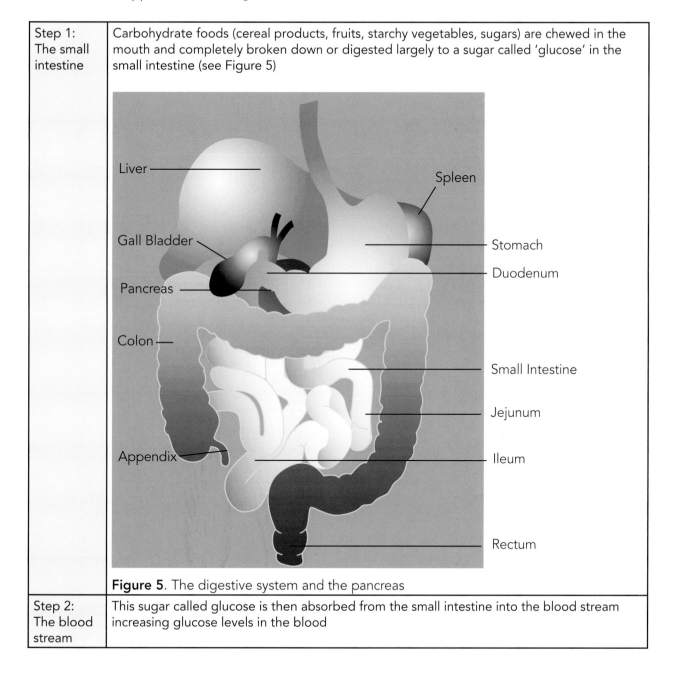 **Figure 5**. The digestive system and the pancreas
Step 2: The blood stream	This sugar called glucose is then absorbed from the small intestine into the blood stream increasing glucose levels in the blood

	No diabetes	Type 1 diabetes	Type 2 diabetes (Lean)	Type 2 diabetes (Overweight or obese)
Step 3 The pancreas	Normally, the rise in blood glucose levels stimulates the pancreas to secrete the hormone 'insulin' into the blood stream.	In Type 1 diabetes the body destroys its own B-cells that produce insulin. This occurs rather suddenly in young people with diabetes. The pancreas stops producing insulin.	In the lean person with Type 2 diabetes, the pancreas secretes less than normal amounts of insulin.	In the overweight person with Type 2 diabetes, even more than normal amounts of insulin could be secreted into the blood stream to compensate for increased resistance to insulin caused by extra fat around the waistline.
Step 4 The muscle cells	'Insulin' circulating in the blood stream acts like a 'key' to 'keyholes' on cells called 'insulin receptors'. It is only then that the glucose doors are opened to allow the transfer of excess glucose in the blood into muscle cells restoring normal levels. It is in muscle cells that glucose is burnt up to produce energy that fuels the body.	Without insulin, blood glucose cannot enter muscle cells resulting in dramatic rises in blood glucose levels.	Because of less than normal amounts of insulin being produced, fewer doors are open for the glucose to enter muscle cells. This results in blood glucose levels higher than normal.	Because of the extra fat around the waistline, the keyholes (insulin receptors) change their shape so that the keys (insulin molecules) do not fit as well and fewer doors are open to allow blood glucose to pass through. These elevated blood sugars cause even more insulin to be secreted by the pancreas into the blood stream. This build-up of insulin and the blockage of its action are known as 'insulin resistance'. With time the pancreas is overworked and gradually tires and fails to produce insulin.

	No diabetes	Type 1 diabetes	Type 2 diabetes (Lean)	Type 2 diabetes (Overweight or obese)
Step 5 The liver	When blood sugars drop with exercise or when we fast, the body also prevents blood glucose levels from dropping too low (less than 4 mmol/l) and causing hypoglycemia. It secretes another hormone from the pancreas called 'glucagon' which causes the liver to offload its storage of glucose (glycogen) restoring blood sugars to within normal levels.	The glycogen stores in the liver are mobilised thus raising blood glucose levels even further.	The glycogen stores in the liver are mobilised thus raising blood glucose levels even further.	The glycogen stores may be mobilised to raise blood glucose levels even further.
Causes of high sugars	In a person with no diabetes, blood sugars remain tightly controlled between 4 and 8 mmol/l because of this balancing act between insulin and glucagon.	Blood sugars are dramatically elevated because the pancreas stops producing insulin and insulin injections are needed for survival.	In Type 2 (lean), blood sugars are elevated largely because the pancreas slowly and gradually stops producing insulin.	In Type 2 (obese) blood sugars are elevated largely because of a tiring pancreas and/or insulin resistance.
Symptoms of high blood sugars	Because blood sugars are closely controlled between 4 and 8 mmol/l there are no symptoms.	•Dramatic onset	•Slow onset •Symptoms can vary from none to mild	•Slow onset •Symptoms can vary from none to mild.
Treatment	None required	Insulin injections plus diet and exercise	•First stage: diet and exercise •Second stage: diet and exercise plus anti-diabetic tablets •Third stage: diet and exercise plus tablets and/or insulin	•First stage: diet (weight loss) and exercise •Second stage: diet and exercise plus anti-diabetic tablets •Third stage: diet and exercise plus tablets and/or insulin

What are the symptoms of insulin resistance and pre-diabetes?

You will usually show no symptoms at all if you have insulin resistance and pre-diabetes, as blood sugars are not high enough. In fact, you may have both conditions for several years without noticing anything. If you have a severe form of insulin resistance you may get dark patches of skin, usually on the back of your neck. This condition is called *acanthosis nigricans*. Other possible sites for these dark patches include elbows, knees, knuckles and armpits. If you have a mild or moderate form of insulin resistance, blood tests may show normal or slightly high blood sugars and high levels of insulin at the same time.

Polycystic Ovary Syndrome (PCOS) is another condition found in 5 to 10 per cent of females in their reproductive years and associated with insulin resistance. Symptoms include irregular menstrual cycles and infertility, masculine hormone secretions resulting in excess hair on the face and body, oily skin and acne. Studies show that 30 to 40 per cent of females with PCOS have pre-diabetes and 7 to 10 per cent have Type 2 diabetes. Weight loss, regular activity and drugs to help improve insulin sensitivity remain the mainstay of treatment. Treatment sometimes also includes hormones to regulate the menstrual cycle and other hormone-related symptoms.

> People with pre-diabetes and PCOS generally show no symptoms of high blood sugars because blood sugar levels are not sufficiently high

What are the common symptoms of high blood sugars in diabetes?

That depends on how abnormally high the blood sugars are. In people with diabetes, symptoms can vary from very mild (Type 2 generally) to dramatic (Type 1) depending on blood sugar levels. The common symptoms of diabetes include:

» Frequent urination (polyuria) as kidneys are forced to get rid of fluid because of changes caused by high blood sugars.

» Unusual thirst (polydipsia) because of lost fluid with excessive urination.

» Excessive drinking to replenish lost fluid. People often drink sweet drinks like soft drinks and juices to alleviate their insatiable thirst—unknowingly aggravating the problem.

» Unusual fatigue because muscle cells are starved of sugar which is normally used as a fuel.

» Unexplained weight loss in those with very high sugars because the body is unable to utilise food. Significant weight loss is uncommon in people with Type 2 diabetes but occurs normally in those with Type 1.

» Blurred vision in some people because the lens of the eye swells because of its high sugar content. This is a temporary situation and does not call for a change of spectacles. As blood glucose levels are stabilised with treatment, blurred vision will improve.

» Ketones in blood and urine, which occurs only in people with Type 1 diabetes with very high blood sugars caused by inadequate insulin or illness. This occurs when the body shifts away from sugars to an alternative source of fuel called ketones which are produced by the fast breakdown of body fat. Ketones include three acids: acetone (what you smell in nail polish), acetoacetate and betahydroxybutyrate. These have an acidic sweet odour that you can smell on people's breath and in their urine. High levels of ketones can result in a serious condition called ketoacidosis and hospitalisation if not appropriately treated.

How do you know if you already have Type 2 diabetes or pre-diabetes?

To screen for Type 2 diabetes you must have a sugar (glucose) test done on blood taken from a vein. Plasma sugar levels can be tested at random (at any time) where a blood sugar level greater than 11millimoles/litre (mmol/l); 198 milligrams/decilitre (mg/dl), indicates the presence of diabetes. Plasma sugar levels can also be tested fasting (after a 10-hour overnight fast) or after you have been challenged with a load of sugar (75 grams of glucose)—a test known as an Oral Glucose Tolerance Test (OGTT).

What is Impaired Fasting Glucose (IFG)?

IFG is an intermediary phase or pre-diabetic state that identifies elevated fasting blood sugar levels (6.1 to 6.9 mmol/l; 110 to 125mg/dl) but not high enough to be classified as diabetes (greater than 7.0 mmol/l; 126 mg/dl). However, since 2003 the American Diabetes Association has used the lower 5.6 (100mg/dl) as the cut-off point. Australians also use this 5.6 cut-off point. The higher fasting blood sugars are within this abnormal range, the higher the risk of developing diabetes in the future.[29] IFG is associated with lower than normal levels of insulin being produced by the pancreas.

Table 3. Blood sugar status determined from a fasting blood sugar test	
Fasting Plasma Glucose (millimoles/litre)	Blood sugar status
≤ 5.6	Normal
Between 5.6 and 6.9	Impaired Fasting Glucose (IFG)
≥ 7.0	Diabetes

What is an Oral Glucose Tolerance Test (OGTT)?

An OGTT is used in individuals with impaired fasting glucose (IFG) to determine their glucose tolerance status. This test assesses how your body reacts when you swallow a concentrated solution of pure sugar (glucose). This is done after an overnight fast and your blood sugars are tested at regular intervals over a two-hour period. Your blood sugar levels at two hours will determine your tolerance level (see Table 4). Levels less than 7.8 mmol/l (140 mg/dl) indicate normal glucose tolerance. Levels greater than 11 (198 mg/dl) indicate the presence of diabetes.

Table 4. Oral Glucose Tolerance Test (blood sugar levels after two hours)	
Plasma sugar level (millimoles/litre)	Blood sugar status
≤ 7.8	Normal
Between 7.8 and 11	Impaired Glucose Tolerance (IGT)
>11	Diabetes

What is Impaired Glucose Tolerance (IGT)?

IGT, like IFG, is an intermediary phase or pre-diabetic state that occurs when the blood sugar levels are higher than normal but not high enough to be diagnosed as diabetes. Those with IGT may show no obvious symptoms because sugars are generally not high enough (see Table 4). A blood sugar level ranging between 7.8 and 11 mmol/l (140 and 198 mg/dl), two hours after being given the sugar solution, indicates that you have IGT and have not been able to handle the glucose load. The higher these two hourly figures are within that abnormal range, the higher the risk of you developing Type 2 diabetes in the future. It has been estimated that 40 per cent of people with IGT with two-hour sugars in the highest range of 9.3 to 11.0 mmol/l (167 to 198 mg/dl) will go on to develop diabetes within five years.[29] IGT most commonly occurs in those with a family history of diabetes, who are overweight, physically inactive and insulin resistant. It has been found that 20 to 35 per cent of people with IFG also have IGT.[30]

Insulin levels in the blood can also be tested after fasting and at the same regular intervals along with blood sugars during an Oral Glucose Tolerance Test to see if you are insulin resistant and to what level. Abnormally high levels of insulin may indicate the presence of insulin resistance, meaning that your pancreas is working overtime trying to maintain normal blood sugars. This could eventually lead to exhausting the pancreas, the result of which would be diabetes.

> People with central obesity who become insulin resistant are more likely to have IGT. People with IGT and/or IFG are in an intermediary or pre-diabetic state and are more likely to develop diabetes and cardiovascular complications in the future if no lifestyle changes are made [31]

3: Our hunter/gatherer ancestors

Historical and anthropological evidence shows hunter/gatherers were generally lean, fit, active and largely free of diseases common in modern societies. They ate food provided as nature packaged it—unrefined, largely unprocessed and high in fibre. These were fresh, lean game, fish, wild berries, tubers and nuts packed with fibre and low in saturated fats, sugars and energy. [32, 33, 34] This is a far cry from what most of us eat today; high energy, low fibre, processed and highly refined foods. In the past 100 years and particularly after the Second World War, there has been a dramatic change in our food supply and eating habits. Remember, the multinational takeaway food chains have only been around for the past 50 years.

> Anthropological evidence shows our ancestral hunter/gatherers to be active, lean and largely free of diseases like diabetes common in Westernised countries today

When the First Fleet landed on Australian shores, it was faced with a very lean hunter-gatherer, the Australian Aborigine. With the adoption of Western food habits (refined sugars, white flour and alcohol etc) and a sedentary lifestyle, indigenous Australians are now facing a much higher incidence of obesity, diabetes and heart disease than other Australians. Alarmingly, this has occurred in a very short period of only 200 years.

Australian Aborigines, like the Pima Indians mentioned earlier, are also thought to have the thrifty gene. Living such a hard, frugal existence, their bodies evolved to be very efficient in using the little food available. This, however, is a liability when faced with a modern, sedentary lifestyle which is why they become obese very quickly and suffer the associated diseases to a much greater extent. In an experiment where a group of urban Australian Aborigines were taken back to the bush to fend for themselves and lead a traditional hunter/gatherer lifestyle again, their health profile improved significantly. [35] Surprisingly, this occurred without any support; no education programs or advice from their doctor, dietitian or nurse educator. Perhaps they were guided by the laws of nature adopted by humans over at least 2.6 million years of evolution.

Are humans more adapted to the hunter/gatherer way of life?

Maybe you, like me, believe in the process of evolution and adaptation to change. Evolution explains how the world and all its beings are not constant, but rather steadily changing and that all organisms (including humans) are transformed in time. Evolution is a time-consuming process that results in heritable changes in a population over long periods of time—hundreds if not thousands of generations. Since the discovery of DNA (the genetic material in our cells) and the study of genetics, *natural selection* or *survival of the fittest* advocated by Darwin in 1859 is now best explained and understood as the adaptation of genes to change. This simply defines evolution but says nothing about whether other forces were helping drive this process. Regardless, humans have been hunter/gatherers for most of our time on earth and hence are better adapted to that way of life. It is only recently that things have dramatically changed and it will take hundreds if not thousands of generations to adapt to our present lifestyle.

It is a basic biological fact that all living organisms survive best on the diet and lifestyle to which they have adapted [32]

What are the stages of human evolution?

Humans have evolved over three distinct historical periods:

1. The **Hunter/Gatherer** or **Paleolithic** period which has accounted for most of our time on earth going back at least 2.6 million years up until the agricultural revolution 10,000 years ago.

Table 5. Stages in the evolution of modern man	
Australopithecus africanus	2.6 million years ago
Homo habilis	1.9 million years ago
Primitive Homo erectus	1.75 million years ago
Homo heidelbergensis	
(Rhodesia Man)	300,000–125,000 years ago
Homo sapiens neanderthalensis	70,000 years ago
Homo sapiens sapiens	
(Cro-Magnon 1)	30,000 years ago
Homo sapiens sapiens	
(Modern Man)	

Anthropological studies have concluded that we lived as hunter/gatherers and that the human genome was largely formed over this period of 104,000 generations (a generation equals 25 years). While unprocessed nuts, tubers and fruit were a major part of the diet, hunted and scavenged lean animal protein was also eaten.

Both hunting and gathering demanded a very high level of activity and energy expenditure

2. The **Agricultural/Peasant** period, with the planting of crops including cereals and the domestication of animals occurred only 10,000 years ago and first started in the Fertile Crescent (Lebanon, Syria, Israel and Turkey) and between the Tigris and the Euphrates rivers in Mesopotamia (modern Iraq). DNA evidence shows very little change in the human genome over this short period of only 400 generations. Humans then started eating more cereals (barley and wheat) and domesticated, as opposed to wild, animals (sheep, cows and goats). While this move resulted in positive changes, the establishment of permanent human settlements, it also resulted in some unfavourable lifestyle changes. Not only did this transition change the diet to more cereal-based products but it also demanded relatively lower levels of activity and energy expenditure compared to that of their Paleolithic hunter/gatherer ancestors.

3. The **Modern/Industrial** period of the past 250 years or only 10 generations. If the change from the Paleolithic period to the agricultural/peasant period had such an impact on human lifestyle, then think of the dramatic changes that have occurred in the modern period when a largely rural population making a living almost entirely from agriculture became an urban society. Also, modern food technology has really changed our food supply dramatically; we are now eating far more refined and processed fats and oils, grain products and sugars than ever before. Furthermore, during this period of increased mechanisation our levels of activity have been seriously reduced. This has been made much worse with the advent of computers and the electronic entertainment media in the past 25 years or one generation.

Socially we are people of the 21st century but genetically we remain citizens of the Paleolithic era [32]

How has our food supply changed in recent times?

What do you think a hunter/gatherer would recognise in today's supermarkets? I suspect nothing other than the fresh produce. Even 100 years ago we had a basic food supply that was based on what we grew. We also had poor nutrition and small body frames, with everyone just trying to survive. Now, we have too much rich food where people are overweight, have high birth weights, diabetes, cardiovascular disease and cancers.

The food industry was rudimentary prior to the Second World War. Since then the whole of agriculture has been transformed as the food industry has responded to the basic tastes that appeal to people: salt, sugar and fat. Today, food processing has become an enormous industry and in the very short period of only two to three generations food technology has provided us with a tremendous range that is being added to daily on our supermarket shelves. We have foods that last on shelves for years without spoiling thanks to a whole range of added preservatives. We have fresh foods like fruits and vegetables which were previously only seasonal and now are available all year round. We have preserved foods, coloured foods, packaged foods, canned foods, frozen foods, dried foods, cured, salted and smoked foods. We are already seeing genetically modified (GM) also known as GE (genetically engineered) foods, the genetic make-up of which has been slightly altered to impart certain favourable qualities. We will soon have a new addition on our shelves—functional foods advertised for their medicinal properties. Food technology today presents us with a dazzling array of colours, flavours, odours, textures, shapes and sizes. The irony of it all is that we have never had so much dietary-related degenerative disease (heart, stroke, cancer, diabetes) as we do today.

> We have never had so much food but, ironically, never so much food-related disease

Perhaps this explains the recent increased demand for basic foods that are organically grown. Maybe our bodies will evolve over future hundreds and thousands of generations to get used to our present food supply, but until then, the price appears to be high; there will inevitably be more degenerative diseases such as diabetes and cardiovascular disease. We need to make some necessary changes now.

4: Type 2 diabetes and the Metabolic Syndrome — prevention and treatment

What is the Metabolic Syndrome?

The 'Metabolic Syndrome' was suspected in the 1950s by a clinician, Jean Vague, in Marseilles, France. This physician noticed that people with central obesity or excess fat around their waistline tended to be more likely to suffer from diabetes and cardiovascular complications. More recently, there has been much scientific interest in this syndrome which is now known to significantly increase the risk of developing diabetes and cardiovascular disease and has become a major public health challenge worldwide. [36, 37]

It has been given different names over the years including *Syndrome* X, *The Deadly Quartet* and *Insulin Resistance Syndrome*. The Metabolic Syndrome affects 20 to 40 per cent of adult populations around the world and is appearing with increasing frequency in children and adolescents. It is believed to be driven by the obesity epidemic. The definition of this syndrome has varied slightly among scientists.[38] However, recently an International Diabetes Federation (IDF) expert group has recommended a practical universal definition to be used worldwide.[39] The Metabolic Syndrome has been defined as central obesity which is thought to be one of the earliest steps and of central importance in the development of the syndrome, [40] plus at least two of any of the following risk factors: high triglycerides, low HDL cholesterol, pre-diabetes, diabetes or high blood pressure (see Figure 6 and Table 6).

Figure 6. Components of the Metabolic Syndrome

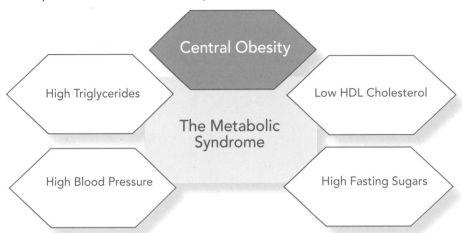

Table 6. The IDF definition of the 'Metabolic Syndrome'

Central obesity–waist circumference*–ethnicity specific (see Table 9)
Plus two or more of the following risk factors:

Raised triglycerides	> 1.7 mmol/l (150 mg/dl) Specific treatment for this abnormality
Reduced HDL cholesterol	< 1.0 mmol/l in men (40 mg/dl) < 1.29 mmol/l in women (50 mg/dl) Specific treatment for this abnormality
Raised Blood Pressure	≥ 130 mm Hg systolic ≥ 85 mm Hg diastolic Treatment of previously diagnosed high blood pressure
Raised fasting plasma glucose	Fasting Plasma Glucose ≥ 5.6mmol/l (100 mg/dl) Previously diagnosed type 2 diabetes

*If Body Mass Index is over 30 kg/m^2, central obesity can be assumed and waist circumference does not need to be measured.

The IDF has also released criteria for the diagnosis in children and adolescents recognising the rapid increase of the syndrome in this age group.[41]

There is obviously a strong association between diabetes and the Metabolic Syndrome since people with Type 2 diabetes generally exhibit a number of the components of this syndrome. Not only do they have high blood sugars, but they are also likely to have central obesity, abnormal blood fats (low HDL cholesterol and high triglycerides) and high blood pressure. Most, but not all people with diabetes would already have the Metabolic Syndrome and these would therefore have the highest risk of cardiovascular disease compared to those with either diabetes or the Metabolic Syndrome alone.[42]

> Most people with diabetes would already have the Metabolic Syndrome

If you have Type 2 diabetes, you must be aware of these other risk factors thought to be behind the 80 per cent of deaths from macrovascular complications and cardiovascular disease in the diabetic population [43,44] (see Table 7).

Table 7. Common Metabolic Syndrome risk factors in diabetes other than high blood sugars

Low HDL (good cholesterol)	<1.29mmol/l (50 mg/dl) in females <1.0 mmol/l (40 mg/dl) in males
High fasting triglycerides	≥1.7 mmol/l (150 mg/dl)
High blood pressure (systolic) (diastolic)	≥ 130 mm Hg ≥ 85 mm Hg
Central obesity (ethnic specific)	(see Table 9)

Common Metabolic Syndrome risk factors in diabetes

As a person with diabetes, your goal first and foremost is to control your blood sugars. However, in order to prevent diabetes vascular complications (heart disease, stroke, peripheral vascular disease) you also need to achieve normal levels of blood fats (LDL cholesterol, HDL cholesterol and triglycerides) and blood pressure. Above all, you need to address the central weight issue, as this is a major underlying problem. Let's look at these factors individually.

1. High blood sugars

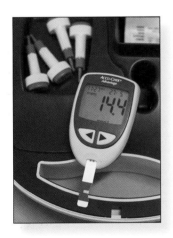

If you have diabetes, blood sugars need to be restored to near normal levels. This should be monitored with a glucometer and reflected in a normal Glycated Haemoglobin (commonly called HbA1c or simply A1C) level of 4 to 6 per cent. Because very strict control is difficult to achieve in diabetes management, a target of less than 7 per cent has generally been used in clinical practice. However, based on new evidence showing reduced complications with even tighter control of blood sugars, this target may have to be lowered.

What is Glycated Haemoglobin (HbA1c)?

This test is done on a sample of blood and reflects your blood sugar levels over the previous two to three months. It is the percentage of haemoglobin in your blood that has sugar attached to it over the lifespan of a red blood cell. The higher the blood sugars over that period, the higher the percentage of haemoglobin that has sugar attached to it. If you think of your home blood sugar test as a single snapshot or photograph, the HbA1c is like a video showing the moment-to-moment average in blood sugars over that period. Reducing blood sugars after meals is now thought to be equally important as reducing fasting blood sugars for achieving HbA1c goals.[45]

Normally when food is eaten, insulin from the pancreas is secreted to bring blood glucose down. It stimulates the conversion of excess glucose to glycogen and its storage in the liver and the muscle. These are very small reserves worth 400 Calories (1673 kilojoules) and 1500 Calories (6276 kilojoules) respectively. On the other hand the body will not let the blood sugars drop too low because the brain needs a constant supply of sugar to function normally. The body does this by secreting another hormone from the pancreas called glucagon that mobilises the above stores of glycogen (glycogenolysis) to raise blood sugars to normal levels. It's a fine balancing act. The brain has first priority and thus has to be supplied with glucose for fuel. This is so important that the body is capable of synthesising glucose from protein in muscle if it has to when glycogen reserves are severely depleted—a process called gluconeogenesis.

> Prior to developing diabetes, your blood sugar levels were finely balanced and kept within normal range at all times by a balancing act of hormones: insulin and glucagon

When you have diabetes, the aim is to maintain sugars within the normal range because low blood sugars (known as hypoglycemia) can cause unpleasant symptoms or in severe cases, fits and coma. These symptoms won't occur if you are treated by diet alone, can occur if you are treated with some diabetic tablets that stimulate your pancreas to secrete more insulin but are most likely to occur if you are treated with insulin.

Table 8. Some symptoms of low blood sugar (hypoglycemia)	
• Intense hunger	• Fast heart beat
• Perspiration	• Confusion and inability to concentrate
• Feeling faint	• Tingling sensation in the mouth and lips
• Fatigue	
• Pallor	

On the other hand, high blood sugars (known as hyperglycemia) can cause damage to small blood vessels in the retina of your eyes, nephrons in your kidneys and nerves in your feet, commonly called microvascular complications. Strict control of blood sugars in diabetes has been shown not only to prevent these microvascular complications [46] but macrovascular complications such as cardiovascular disease as well.[47] The higher blood sugars are the higher the risk of cardiovascular disease.[48]

How does exposure to high blood sugars cause this damage to cells?

The mechanism remains unknown. However, three major theories have been proposed to explain how high blood sugars lead to these chronic complications.[49] One hypothesis is that increased levels of glucose lead to the formation of linkages with proteins forming abnormal substances called advanced glycated end products (AGEs) that cause cell damage. Another theory is based on the observation that high blood sugars increase glucose conversion to sorbitol, which is also known to lead to dysfunction of cells. Finally, oxidative stress and the generation of free radicals are thought to be involved in the development of these microvascular complications.

> If you have diabetes, aim to keep your blood sugars within the range of 4 to 8 mmoles/litre. Strict blood glucose control has been shown to prevent these complications.

2. Abnormal blood fats

As shown already, insulin is a hormone that has profound effects on your blood sugars. However, it also has important effects on your blood fats. A high level of insulin (hyperinsulinemia) caused by insulin resistance:

> » **Promotes the synthesis of fat in the liver.** As glycogen stores in the liver reach saturation levels, extra glucose in the blood is taken up by liver cells to make the fat—triglycerides. This in turn results in lowering levels of the good HDL cholesterol.

» **Inhibits breakdown of fat stores in your body.** This makes it harder for you to lose weight.

People with Type 2 diabetes generally have higher triglycerides and lower good HDL cholesterol levels than normal as part of their Metabolic Syndrome risk profile, [50, 51] which could significantly increase their risk of cardiovascular disease. [52, 53, 54] High intakes of carbohydrate resulting in even higher blood sugars can exacerbate this problem even further.

> The most common blood fat abnormalities in Type 2 diabetes are elevated triglycerides and low HDL cholesterol

Population studies have also shown that a high proportion of adults with Type 2 diabetes, like people without diabetes of the same middle age, have high cholesterol levels. Also their LDL cholesterol (bad cholesterol) is high but not significantly higher than it is in those with no diabetes. What is different, however, is the structure of this bad cholesterol. LDL cholesterol particles in people with diabetes are smaller and denser and are much more damaging.[55]

> The bad LDL cholesterol particles in people with Type 2 diabetes are usually smaller and denser than normal which makes them more damaging in terms of blocking arteries

These combined blood fat abnormalities (low HDL, high triglycerides and small dense LDL cholesterol) may explain the higher rate of heart disease and stroke in people with diabetes. It is also interesting to note that these abnormalities are already present early on in people who do not have diabetes but are in the pre-diabetes stage, even more of a reason to implement some lifestyle changes early on in those at risk.

These abnormal blood fats in people with Type 2 diabetes, along with high blood sugars, blood pressure and smoking, cause blockage of large blood vessels leading to heart attack, stroke and ulcers and gangrene of the feet.

On average, if you have diabetes you have a much higher risk of heart disease and stroke and other large blood vessel diseases (ulcers) and for this reason, need to be even more aware of your blood fat levels.[56, 57] All it takes is a fasting blood test with your general practitioner to find out what your blood fats are like.

Many people with diabetes are unaware of the fact that cardiovascular disease is a complication of diabetes. A survey carried out by the American Heart Association showed that only one third of people with diabetes considered heart disease to be a serious complication of the disease, yet two thirds had already experienced some form of heart problem.

Changing your diet, introducing some regular exercise, losing some of that extra weight can all help control your blood sugars, which in turn can help correct some of these blood fat abnormalities.

> I would strongly recommend that all people with diabetes and abnormal blood fats seek professional dietary advice from a qualified dietitian experienced in diabetes management

If correcting blood sugar levels with diet, lifestyle measures and diabetic tablets fail to correct your blood fats your doctor may start you on medications to:

» **Lower your bad LDL cholesterol:** Statins are a class of drugs that stop your body from making cholesterol. They are generally the first line of treatment for lowering LDL cholesterol in people with diabetes. They include drugs such as Atorvastatin (Lipitor™), Simvastatin (Lipex™), Pravastatin (Pravachol™), Rosuvastatin (Crestor™).[58] Several recent large-scale studies have shown, and continue to show, that lowering LDL cholesterol with these drugs significantly reduces the chance of cardiovascular disease whether you have diabetes or not.[59, 60, 61, 62]

> In people with diabetes, the target is to lower LDL cholesterol to 2.5 mmol/l (100 mg/dl) or less

Some people cannot tolerate statins because of side effects such as muscle ache and soreness. These people are generally given another class of drugs that work not on inhibiting the synthesis of cholesterol by the body, but by inhibiting the absorption of cholesterol from the small intestine. These include drugs like Ezetimibe (Ezetrol™) and generally are not as effective as statins.

» **Lower your triglycerides and raise good HDL cholesterol**: People with diabetes still have high residual cardiovascular risk even after statin therapy largely because this class of drugs does not address the Metabolic Syndrome risk factors of high triglycerides and low HDL cholesterol commonly found in this group. Even high-dose statin therapy was unable to sufficiently improve clinical outcomes in people with diabetes, as demonstrated in the TNT study.[63]

> In people with diabetes the target is to raise HDL cholesterol to 1.0 mmol/l (40 mg/dl) or more and to lower triglycerides to 1.7 mmol/l (150 mg/dl) or less

Thus, some people with diabetes are in need of therapy in addition to statins to achieve adequate improvement in the risk of cardiovascular disease. This can be achieved by using other classes of drugs called fibrates such as Fenofibrate (Lipidil™) or Gemfibrozil (Lopid™) which significantly lower triglycerides and raise HDL cholesterol[64, 65, 66] and Omega 3 fatty acids (fish oils) which have also been shown to significantly reduce triglycerides in people with coronary heart disease and high triglycerides but have no effect on HDL cholesterol.[67]

Combination drug therapy

A combination of statins and fibrates has been tested on people without diabetes with very positive effects on all blood fats and a major positive effect of raising HDL cholesterol. There are studies going on at present to investigate the effects of this combination therapy specifically in people with Type 2 diabetes. By the end of this decade, data should shed more light on their safety and efficacy. Until then, this combination of drugs is unlikely to be widely used.

The addition of the vitamin niacin (nicotinic acid) to statin therapy has also been tested with significant improvements in all blood fat levels in people with coronary heart disease.[69]

Side effects to cholesterol lowering drugs

The side effects to statins include mild to severe muscle ache and soreness and both statins and fibrates can result in abnormal liver function tests. The most common side effects to niacin include flushing, characterised by redness, warmth and itching. These side effects should be closely monitored by your doctor for some time after starting drugs for any necessary change of dose or type of medication.

3. Overweight and obesity

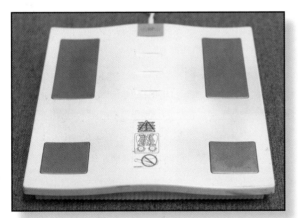

Humans have evolved to efficiently store any extra food for a rainy day in the form of fat (triglycerides) in what is called adipose tissue or fat stores. Adipose tissue is not uniformly distributed throughout the body, with 80 per cent of all body fat normally stored under the skin (subcutaneous fat). The other major fat—containing depot is the central waistline, or visceral fat compartment where fat is stored deep down, which makes up around 10 per cent of all body fat.[70] Some people have a tendency to store more around their waistline than others and it seems to run in families. These fat stores have several important functions in the body:

> » Fat acts as the largest reserve of potential energy in your body. Your body can draw on this enormous reserve in case of prolonged physical activity, during breastfeeding, during dieting and starvation. Remember, human beings as hunter/gatherers were subjected to extremes of feasts and famines.

» Fat under the skin acts as insulation material especially to conserve heat, otherwise you would have to wear much heavier clothes particularly in colder climates.

» Fats (triglycerides) can be formed from sugars in the blood, thus protecting the body from toxic levels of high sugars commonly found in people with badly controlled diabetes.

» Fat can be used for emergency brain fuel by converting to ketones when blood sugar levels drop too low for long periods.

» Fat stores have recently been found to secrete a number of substances (for example, leptin and adiponectin) that play an important role in controlling appetite, energy metabolism and insulin resistance in people with excess body fat.

So, fat reserves in the form of triglycerides have an important role to play in your body. However, excessive fat may have some serious consequences. The average 70 kilogram (154 lb) man has around 10 kilograms (22 lbs) of fat reserves worth 90,000 Calories (376,560 kilojoules). This constitutes around 14 per cent of body weight—the normal range in males is 12 to 17 per cent. Normal weight females average 19 to 25 per cent so they have more body fat than males—6 to12 per cent of this is the essential body fat that females need for normal body function. In morbidly obese people, this store may be much larger and form up to 70 per cent of body weight. Weight loss from these body fat stores is an important goal for all overweight and obese people who have, or are at risk of, diabetes.[71]

As mentioned earlier, if you are at increased risk, losing even 5 to10 per cent of body weight can, in most cases, delay the onset of or prevent diabetes. This, initially, may be a reasonable goal to aim for. If you already have diabetes, this moderate weight loss can also reduce insulin resistance, decrease fasting blood sugar concentrations and reduce the need for diabetes medications. The improvement in blood sugars is directly related to the percentage of weight lost; marked weight loss (20 to 30 per cent of body weight) following gastrointestinal surgery has been shown to normalise blood sugars in up to two thirds of obese people with Type 2 diabetes.[72] A patient of mine who was a competitor on a TV weight-loss reality show had recently lost over 70 kilograms (40 per cent of his body weight) by the time he was referred to me, a major loss indeed. Admittedly, this was achieved with several hours of exercise a day and a dramatic change in diet. He used to be on both insulin and blood sugar tablets to control his blood sugars and now, because of the dramatic weight loss, requires neither. He is now on a healthy diet alone and achieves excellent blood sugar control.

Weight loss, particularly from around the waistline, has important additional health benefits if you have diabetes. It improves other Metabolic Syndrome risk factors by decreasing blood pressure and reversing blood fat abnormalities (a decrease in small dense LDL cholesterol particles, a decrease in triglycerides and an increase in HDL cholesterol) thus reducing the risk of cardiovascular complications.

> Weight loss, particularly from the waistline area, reduces insulin resistance, improves fasting blood sugars and other Metabolic Syndrome risk factors

Apples versus pears

Studies support the view that it is not only the total percentage of body fat, but also where the fat sits on the body that is important to health. If you have 'central obesity', you are more likely to have metabolic syndrome risk factors.[73, 74] This is more commonly known as the 'apple shape' form of obesity usually found in men.

On the other hand, the type of fat distribution most common in women is of low risk and often described as 'pear shape' where the fat deposits are mainly found under the skin in the lower parts of the body (buttocks, hips and thighs). The high-risk central 'apple shape' obesity, common in men, is also seen in many women after menopause. Scientists believe that visceral fat that accumulates deep in the waistline area is metabolised differently from fat located directly under the skin and in other parts of the body and this difference contributes to the risks of diabetes and the Metabolic Syndrome.[75, 36]

Figure 7. The two shapes of obesity—apples versus pears

MEN

WOMEN

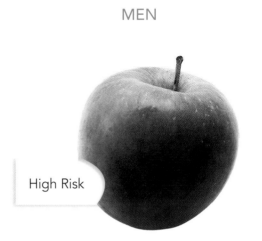

High Risk

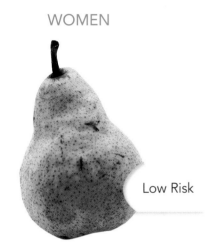

Low Risk

How is 'central obesity' measured?

Special imaging tests such as MRIs (Magnetic Resonance Imaging) and CT (Computed Tomography) scans are used to map the distribution of fat in the waistline area—how

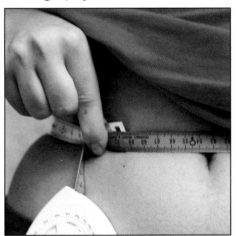

much is under the skin (subcutaneous) and how much is stored deep (visceral).[76] However, simply measuring your waist circumference correctly gives us a good idea. The healthy cut-off points for different ethnic groups are shown in Table 9 based on data available at this time. The International Diabetes Federation (IDF) Consensus Group agreed upon these figures in 2005. It is also recommended that ethnic group specific cut-off points be used for people of the same ethnic group wherever they are living.

Table 9. IDF[†] ethnic specific values for waist circumference (as measure of central obesity). Waist circumference in centimetres (inches).

Ethnic Group	Male		Female
Europids*	≥ 94	(37.0 in)	≥ 80 (31.5 in)
South Asians	≥ 90	(35.4 in)	≥ 80 (31.5 in)
Chinese	≥ 90	(35.4 in)	≥ 80 (31.5 in)
Japanese	≥ 85	(33.5 in)	≥ 90 (35.4 in)
Ethnic South/Central Americans	≥ 90	(35.4 in)	≥ 80 (31.5 in)
Sub-Saharan Africans	≥94	(37.0 in)	≥ 80 (31.5 in)
Eastern Mediterranean and Middle East (Arab) populations	≥ 94	(37.0 in)	≥ 80 (31.5 in)

[†]International Diabetes Federation
* In the USA, Adult Treatment Panel III values (102 cm , 40 in males; 88 cm, 34.6 in females) are used for clinical purposes
Reproduced with permission from IDF (www.idf.org)

Battle of the bulge

By and large, being overweight or obese was and still is unheard of in traditional hunter/gatherer societies. The reason is simple: plenty of exercise and a frugal low-calorie diet. Obesity remained a rarity up until the Industrial Revolution in the 18th century and was confined to the upper classes and commonly viewed as a status symbol. Since then, with the escalation of obesity, gluttony has been restored to its status as a deadly sin where it has remained ever since.

Diets with different percentages of protein, fat and carbohydrate have come and gone and the problem gets worse. These include:

» **Very Low Carbohydrate Diets.** An example is the very popular Dr Atkins Diet Revolution.[77] These diets are very low in carbohydrate in the initial phase, very high in protein and very high in fat, particularly saturated animal fat, as people are allowed to eat as much dairy and meat fats as they want. This type of diet is not new and was first proposed as far back as 1864. It has resurfaced every decade since the 1950s. The recommended intake for dietary protein for adults is around 0.75 grams per kilogram of body weight per day. These high-protein diets advocate up to 4 grams per kilogram of body weight, which is far in excess of what your body needs. Restricting protein has been found to effectively slow the progression of kidney disease in diabetic and non-diabetic patients, [78, 79, 80] which makes these diets a problem and also excess protein can result in the excretion of calcium from your body, decreasing bone strength and predisposing you to osteoporosis.

> Not recommended for people with diabetes: unbalanced, too low in carbohydrates and fibre, too extreme and too high in the bad fats. Excess dietary protein can potentially cause kidney disease—a major complication of diabetes.

» **Very Low Fat Diets.** An example is Dr Ornishs' diet.[81] This diet is very low in fat and protein and very high in carbohydrate.

> Not recommended for people with diabetes: too extreme in carbohydrate (glycemic) load

» **Diabetic associations/Heart Foundation Diet.** This conventional diet is moderate in carbohydrate, moderate in fat and adequate in lean protein. It has been recommended for over 25 years by associations around the world.

> Diet recommended for people with diabetes. It is balanced and addresses cardiovascular risk factors as saturated fats are kept to a low of 8 per cent.

» **Lower Carbohydrate Higher Protein Diets.** More recently The CSIRO Total Well Being Diet [82, 83, 84] varies slightly from the Diabetic Association/Heart Foundation Diet in that carbohydrate intake is slightly reduced and protein is doubled.

May be suitable for people with diabetes on proviso that no osteoporosis or early signs of kidney disease are present

The hunter/gatherer diet

Our ancestors ate diets that varied in their composition, depending on availability. Diets were generally high in protein, moderate in glycemic load from unprocessed unrefined carbohydrate from fruits and vegetables and tubers, moderate in fat but low in saturated fats. Most importantly, their intake of calories would have been low compared to their output of energy due to the fact that both gathering and hunting are both intricately associated with high activity levels.[32]

The overwhelming majority of people lose weight initially on all these diets and keep it off for a year because their caloric intake is reduced, only to regain what they have lost in the long term. This is because the emotional reasons for overeating are not addressed, the diets are often unbalanced, unhealthy and hard to comply with, and because acquired bad eating habits are hard to break. More importantly, most don't involve enough movement to help this weight-loss process become a long-term solution.

Why starve when you can take a pill?

Some people have given up trying with diets and have resorted to drugs to solve their problem, the old Passive Patient Syndrome again. At best this is a short-term solution to a lifelong problem. In the early 19th century doctors began prescribing thyroid compounds that stimulate metabolism to help weight loss. Then there was Human Chorionic Gonadotrophin (HCG), a hormone which was popular in spite of having no effect on weight. Next up was Fen-Phen, a combination of two drugs that increase metabolism which was taken off the market because of some serious side effects. Still with us today is a new generation of drugs like Reductil™ that reduces appetite and Xenical™, a drug that partly inhibits the digestion and absorption of dietary fats, the side effects of which include fatty stools and oily discharge from the anus.

If all else fails resort to the knife

Weight-loss surgery is now becoming more popular. Operations like gastric staples, bands and sleeves to limit stomach capacity and bowel bypass surgery, where the length of the small intestine is shortened to reduce absorption of food, are now being performed as a last resort in morbidly obese people. Liposuction, which involves the insertion of a cannula to extract aesthetic fat deposits from under the skin, not in the intra abdominal area where it counts for Metabolic Syndrome risk factors, is now one of the most common cosmetic surgeries performed.

   Unfortunately, we are losing the battle of the bulge in spite of a billion-dollar weight loss industry including low-fat foods, low-carbohydrate foods, weight-loss salons, health clubs, cosmetic surgery and drugs.

What can you do?

The formula for long-term weight loss is simple: **Eat Less** (reduce energy intake) **Move More** (increase energy expenditure); yet people still do not seem to understand. I often use a simple analogy to help explain weight loss. If I compare your weight to your bank account, a reduction in your balance will definitely occur if you withdraw more than you deposit. It is a simple formula. If the amount of money you withdraw always exceeds the total amount deposited, irrespective of the size of the denominations, your bank balance will simply disappear in due course. Similarly, weight loss is bound to occur when your expenditure of calories through your metabolism and physical activity exceeds your energy intake from food. If you treated your body the way you treated your bank account, you would definitely lose weight.

   The message is simple: spend more with regular physical activity and take in fewer calories by eating more leafy vegetables which are very low in calories (equivalent to 5 cent coins) instead of the complex carbohydrate foods ($20 notes), protein foods ($50 notes), fats, alcohol and refined carbohydrates ($100 notes).

   It's also a matter of balance. You don't have to cut anything out of your diet completely, but get your proportions right: plenty of greens, moderate amounts of low-GI carbohydrate and protein and limited amounts of fats, sugars and alcohol (see the Healthy Food Pyramid Figure 9, page 93).

The diet should be reduced in calories if necessary but also balanced to meet your nutrient requirements and take into account principles to control blood sugars, blood pressure and blood fats

Setting realistic goals

You should also set yourself some realistic short and long-term goals when trying to lose weight. Setting small and achievable goals (for example half to one kilogram/1 to 2 pounds per week) allows you to experience success, which can be used as a foundation for additional lifestyle alterations. Strategies such as self behaviour monitoring (keeping records of food and physical activity), avoiding triggers that prompt eating and identifying barriers and ways to overcome them can support this process. Do not expect to return to the weight you were in your late teens. Setting unrealistic goals is disheartening, in most cases unachievable and above all unnecessary. Initially, aim to lose 5 to 10 per cent of your body weight. Aesthetically, this might not meet your expectations but you would be surprised what difference it makes to all the risk factors and your need for diabetes tablets.

An initial realistic goal to aim for if you are overweight is to lose 5 to 10 per cent of your body weight

Using scales or waistline measurements?

Remember, medically, it is the central obesity that is the major problem and, as long as your waistline is shrinking and you are pulling that belt in gradually, you are well and truly on track. This is important because body composition changes may occur without showing much of a change on the scales particularly if you are exercising regularly. This is due to an increase in body muscle (which weighs more than fat) and a corresponding decrease in body fat.

You should monitor progress not only by the scales but more importantly by changes in your waistline measurements

4. Hypertension or high blood pressure

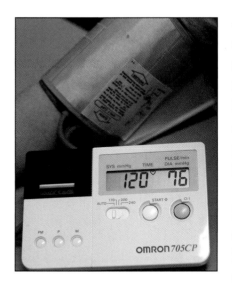

Approximately 50 per cent of people with Type 2 diabetes have high blood pressure and it needs to be addressed to prevent long-term complications[85]. This may even exist prior to the diagnosis of the disease. High blood pressure puts you at increased risk of damage to large and small blood vessels. In clinical practice, ideal blood pressure is less than 130 systolic/85 diastolic.

Positive steps must be taken to treat or control high blood pressure. Adopting healthy lifestyle measures is extremely important in managing this. These include weight loss if necessary, moderating the amount of alcohol and giving up smoking.

Reducing the amount of salt in the diet often helps too. There is no evidence that humans undertook salt extraction before the Agricultural Revolution 10,000 years ago. However, in the Western diet, the average person consumes a high intake of around 10 grams per day. The huge majority of this intake is derived from salt added to foods by food manufacturers or from salt added at the table. Only 10 per cent of the salt we eat today comes from natural foodstuffs so salt is a relative newcomer to the human diet. To reduce salt in your diet, you will need to reduce your consumption of processed foods.

Taking regular aerobic activity, for example low to moderate intensity activities such as walking, helps to lower blood pressure. Exercise does this by improving blood flow to the heart and increasing the flexibility of arteries.

In many cases, medication is needed in addition to these lifestyle changes to control blood pressure. However it is done, make sure your blood pressure is well controlled to help prevent complications.

Make sure your blood pressure is well controlled at 130/85 or less to prevent heart disease, stroke and eye and kidney damage

What can you do to prevent long-term complications of diabetes and the Metabolic Syndrome?

Scientific evidence has shown that you can reduce the long-term complications of diabetes and the Metabolic Syndrome, and that is good news. Controlling blood sugars alone can certainly reduce damage to your eyes, kidneys and nerves in your feet. However, this alone does not protect you from the debilitating cardiovascular complications of heart disease, stroke, foot ulcers and gangrene. Medical specialists, both diabetes and cardiovascular, agree that you also need to control your blood fats, blood pressure and work on losing some weight off that waistline. A change in lifestyle is the cornerstone to managing this problem or preventing it in the first place.

Table 10. Targets you need to achieve to reduce long-term diabetes complications

HbA1c *	< 7.0	
LDL cholesterol	< 2.5 mmol/l	100 mg/dl
HDL cholesterol	> 1.0 mmol/l	40 mg/dl
Triglycerides	< 1.7 mmol/l	150 mg/dl
Systolic Blood Pressure	< 130 mm Hg	
Diastolic Blood Pressure	< 85 mm Hg	
Weight loss	5–10% of body weight if overweight	

* An index of blood sugar control over the past 2 to 3 months

PART 2:

Lifestyle management of diabetes and the Metabolic Syndrome

In Westernised countries today, we commonly suffer from what has been referred to as Passive Patient Syndrome a giving up of personal responsibility for our health. Our reliance on modern medicine, doctors and drugs, has made us less inclined to take care of ourselves to help our body defend itself from health threats like Type 2 diabetes and cardiovascular disease.

Most people I see in our diabetes clinic rely on a number of drugs to control their blood sugars, blood pressure, cholesterol and triglycerides. More recently, some are now taking new generation drugs to help them lose weight. The pharmaceutical industry is now looking at developing the poly-pill, a cocktail of many of these drugs which has been promised to be the wonder drug of the future. However, it is important to take some responsibility in treating, or better still preventing these diseases by making some changes to your eating habits and levels of activity.

Natural nutrition is your real medicine. Since your entire body is made from nutrients that you obtain from food, primary health care cannot rest with synthetic drugs and medical technology alone. What and how much you eat and drink and how your food is processed and cooked all have a bearing on your diabetes control. [86] Your other important medicine is exercise, which is equally important in preventing and treating diabetes and its Metabolic Syndrome risk factors.[87, 88]

> Your weapons for the prevention and/or treatment of Type 2 diabetes lie not with drugs alone, but with your knives, forks and walking shoes

In Westernised countries the situation is serious. In Australia only 5 per cent of the adult population meet both the recommended leisure time activity and fruit and vegetables needed for good health [89] 'Physical inactive Australian adults are costing the health care system 1.5 billion dollars' [90]. In the US it was estimated way back in 1990 that the health care cost of chronic diseases was two thirds of a trillion dollars and affected 90 million Americans.[91] That was alarming, but today this figure would be much higher with the aging of the baby boomer generation. It has been estimated that one half of deaths in the United States result from preventable causes and that 28 per cent of these preventable deaths are caused by a combination of unhealthy diets and physical inactivity.[92]

What lifestyle changes can you make to help control diabetes and its Metabolic Syndrome risk factors?

Confusion prevails as to what lifestyle changes you need to make and this may be because you are constantly bombarded with contradictory nutrition information in the media. Add to this the array of processed refined and takeaway food and it's no wonder you have problems. In Australia, even back in the eighties, 35 to 40 per cent of the household budget was spent on food cooked outside the home. This figure is likely to be much higher today. In the United States today, units are now being built without fully equipped kitchens. The food preparation areas are called kitchenettes and are equipped with the bare minimum; a fridge, a sink and a microwave oven. Maybe the worse is yet to come!

The answer is simple. Nature itself, through a slow and long process of evolution has laid down the rules. Your body evolved to move, to take in certain foods, in a certain form and in a certain way to stay healthy. We, today, have simply broken some of these rules with our energy saving devices, our food technology and processing techniques.

In order to change lifestyle behaviours, you need to know what to do first. I would like to take you on an imaginary trip 'back to basics' as a hunter/gatherer to explain the necessary lifestyle changes you can make. The basic principles are simple and can be explained easily.

> Knowing what to do is the first step to changing behaviours

As mentioned in Chapter 4, you are likely to present with a number of risk factors when diagnosed with diabetes. Going 'back to basics' with food and exercise often helps control all of these.

> Going back to basics helps control all your Metabolic Syndrome risk factors of diabetes

Figure 8. Lifestyle-related 'Metabolic Syndrome' risk factors in diabetes

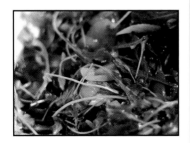

High sugars

High Cholesterol

Low HDL

High Triglycerides

High Blood Pressure

Central Obesity

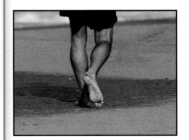

Let's take a trip, pick up some of nature's tips and cut through some of the myths, misconceptions and confusion you could be facing today.

Small changes can result in major health benefits

Picture yourself back as a hunter/gatherer again. Not a pleasant thought because now you don't have the luxury of choices. No more buttons to push, no more cars to ride, no access to processed foods and certainly no lining up at the Golden Arches for a quick 1000 calorie (4184 kilojoule) meal. The first thing you need to do just to survive is find food and water. You will not have the luxury of running water or fridges. By the end of three months your diabetes will undoubtedly improve with weight loss, better blood sugars, blood pressure and blood fats. That is if you survive!

5: The Lifestyle Factor — Activity

While we Westerners sit and press buttons for several hours a day or drive up to the Golden Arches and get a 1000 Calorie (4184 kilojoule) meal in a matter of minutes, a female of the Indians of the Amazon has to dig for hours to get enough tubers to feed her family for the next meal. Populations living in deserts, the Arctic or similar marginal places can spend several hours a day hunting or gathering.

> Food in hunter/gatherer societies has always been intricately related to high activity levels

Physical activity in today's sedentary societies is far lower than that of our hunter/gatherer ancestors.[93] Human activity levels have gradually dropped since the hunter/gatherer period through the time of the Agricultural Revolution and certainly during the Industrial Revolution period through to today (see Chapter 3). A major drop has occurred in the past century for the following reasons:

» Probably the blame mostly lies with the invention of the motor car. We all spend an hour or more a day driving a car where we would otherwise be walking.
» Work used to be active but is now largely mechanised and we spend time sitting in front of a monitor pressing buttons instead.
» We used to climb stairs, now we use escalators or elevators.
» We used to push lawn mowers, now these machines are automated.
» We used to rake our yards, now we use an electric blower.
» We used to wash our clothes by hand, now we have washing machines.
» We used to handwash our dishes, now we use a dish washer.
» We used to spend time washing our cars, now we run them through an automated car wash.

- » We used to walk our golf courses, now we use a buggy.
- » We used to manually brush our teeth, now we use an electric tooth brush.
- » Our kids used to walk or cycle to school, now they are driven.
- » Schools generally dedicate a minimum amount of time to physical activity and sports.
- » Our kids used to spend hours playing ball in the streets after school, now they can't wait to sit in front of their Nintendo or Play Station for hours while munching on high-calorie snack foods like chocolate or salted chips.
- » If any of our kids show any desire to move, they are diagnosed as 'hyperactive' and put on drugs to slow them down!

Unlike what we see in hunter/gatherer societies, for many of us in developed countries, both work hours and leisure time are characterised by lack of activity. Studies have shown that this sedentary way of life increases the risk of diabetes even without a weight problem. There is plenty of evidence supporting the hypothesis that physical activity, along with other dietary therapies, may delay or even prevent the onset of Type 2 diabetes in patients at risk [94].

> Lack of activity is now recognized as a risk in itself for developing diabetes

Hunter/gatherers, whose food is rather low in calories and who are very active, are normally very lean. Today, most of us gradually gain weight from the time we are in our twenties or earlier. This phenomenon of weight gain with age, is not generally seen in hunter/gatherer populations who remain rather active all their lives.

What is physical activity?

Physical activity has been defined as 'bodily movement produced by the contraction of muscle that requires energy to be spent over and above what your body would spend resting'.[87] I would like to compare your body to a car at this stage to help you understand this concept. Being sedentary is like your car while switched on but not moving, burning fuel but not much. Driving your car or accelerating is like exercising, increasing activity and burning up more fuel. While your car burns petrol as a source of fuel, your body burns both sugars and fats. During continuous moderate exercise, energy is derived mainly from the breakdown of the body's stores of fat and carbohydrate.

There are mainly two broad categories of activity or exercise:

> » **Aerobic activity** consists of rhythmic, repeated and continuous movement of the same large muscle groups for at least 10 minutes at a time. These muscle groups mainly include leg and arm muscles. These exercises improve your fitness level and include walking, jogging (including treadmills), swimming, cycling, rowing and using step machines commonly found in gyms. If you push yourself hard enough you will find yourself having to breathe harder, hence the name aerobic activity. If performed at least three times a week over a period of many weeks, these aerobic exercises can improve your cardiovascular fitness level.
> » **Resistance exercise** consists of activities that use muscle strength to move a weight or work against a resistance load. Examples include weight lifting and exercise using weight machines in gyms. These exercises mainly increase muscle mass and strength.

Health authorities recommend both forms of exercise for patients with Type 2 diabetes. Resistance exercise has been found to be as effective as aerobic exercise in improving insulin sensitivity.[95]

> Health authorities recommend both aerobic activity and resistance training for people with diabetes

The human body is a machine equipped with the perfect apparatus to move and adapt to regular physical activity; the right muscles, bones, joints, tendons, ligaments, a way of delivering oxygen to exercising muscles (haemoglobin in the red blood cells) and enzymes in muscles that help metabolise or burn fat and sugar. That means if you are very unfit today and start out with a regular aerobic exercise like walking (3–5 times per week for at least 30 minutes), your body will adapt to that regular regime to become fit within eight to ten weeks. It does so by increasing oxygen uptake in the lungs, increasing oxygen carrying capacity by raising haemoglobin levels in the blood and raising levels of certain enzymes in the muscle needed to aerobically metabolise fuel.

Today, having done no exercise for a long time, your body is like a badly tuned car, accelerate and there will be plenty of smoke coming out of that exhaust. This is because the air and fuel are not mixed in the right proportions. Similarly, when you start out with your programme you might have pain in your muscles the next day caused by increased concentrations of lactic acid, a result of not being able to burn your fuel (fat and sugar) aerobically. In eight to ten weeks your body will adapt and become like a well-tuned racing car that performs at its best with very little, if any, smoke emerging from that exhaust.

> The human body is perfectly equipped for and can adapt to regular physical activity

Getting started with your exercise program

Before beginning a serious physical activity program more vigorous than brisk walking, you should be assessed by your doctor. Age, cardiovascular risk and other factors (for example, mobility problems, arthritis and other joint problems, respiratory problems from smoking) will determine what exercise is safe for you. There are other issues about exercise and diabetes that you should be aware of. These include:

» Foot care because of the potential problems with circulation and nerve damage.
» The issue of increased risk of hypoglycemia (low blood sugars) in patients on insulin and certain diabetic medications.
» Chronic badly controlled blood sugars (greater than 10 mmol/l most of the time) need to be addressed by adjusting the dose of blood sugar tablets if need be, as exercise potentially can raise blood sugars even further under

these abnormal metabolic circumstances.

» If treated by insulin, the presence of ketones in your blood indicates bad diabetes control and this definitely needs to be addressed by increasing your insulin dose before embarking on your new exercise program. At this stage you most likely would not be feeling well enough to do any serious exercise anyway.

> Get medical clearance from your doctor before starting your serious exercise regime

It is probably not a bad time to buy a pedometer to see how many steps you take on your average day. This will give you a baseline on which to build.

What type of physical activity did your ancestors do as hunter/gatherers?

Your ancestors engaged in various forms of physical activity and they did that daily just to survive. They had no choice. Although they jumped, carried, climbed, stretched and leaped as they protected themselves and foraged and hunted for food, their main form of physical activity was walking and running. In fact they walked or ran an estimated 8 to 16 kilometres a day.[93] They did what we call today a combination of aerobics (walking and running) and resistance training such as carrying water, game and wood back to camp. You should also do both aerobic activity and resistance training as they both have benefits in managing diabetes.

> In performing their daily chores, your ancestral hunter/gatherers had to do both aerobic and resistance exercise just to survive

In hunter/gatherer and traditional societies, physical activity was and still remains a necessity not a choice. Given the options of hunting/gathering or pressing buttons and driving cars I believe most would choose the latter. However, knowing how important physical activity is to diabetes control and overall health today, I believe we must change or face the consequences.

Physical activity in ancestral hunter/gatherer societies was a necessity not a choice

The effects of physical activity on Metabolic Syndrome risk factors in diabetes

A recent systematic review of reliable data available on the benefits of exercise in people with Type 2 diabetes clearly shows that exercise, independent of diet, helps regulate blood sugar levels, increases insulin sensitivity, and decreases blood fats while burning up body stores of fat—helping them to lose weight at the same time.[88]

1. The effect of physical activity on your blood sugar levels

Patients who exercised regularly were found to significantly drop their two to three months average of blood sugars (HbA1c) by 30 per cent which is comparable to what you would expect from prescribed blood sugar tablets [88] and this effect has also been found to be independent of weight loss.[96] Such improvement is likely to reduce small blood vessel damage or complications such as damage to retinas, kidneys and neurons.

What would happen to your blood sugars if you walked regularly?
Well, assuming your blood sugars are reasonably controlled, you feel well and have no ketones in your urine (for people with Type 1 diabetes on insulin), they would drop. Sugar is the fuel that your body burns up with every step that you take. It's like the petrol in that tank. The little furnaces in each of your muscle cells called mitochondria start working overtime to burn the sugar to meet your energy needs. What a natural way to bring your blood sugars down! Regular physical activity not only burns up blood sugars directly but also improves insulin sensitivity; it helps your insulin transfer sugar from your blood stream into muscle and fat cells.[95]

> Regular exercise improves insulin sensitivity in muscles and significantly improves blood sugar control

You might want to experiment with checking your blood sugars before and after a 30 to 45 minute session of walking. You might be pleasantly surprised to see your blood sugars drop. Imagine if you had to walk for several hours a day as your ancestors did.

Have you seen the Peter Weir thriller *Witness* set among the Amish of Pennsylvania, USA? They're people who were persecuted in Europe for their religious beliefs and migrated to the United States for religious freedom in the early 1700s. They are a tight community and for that reason have remained fairly isolated genetically from the rest of the American population. They have also rejected our modern way of life. Even today they basically live very much like they did 250 years ago in Europe. The Amish don't use any modern conveniences; they don't have any electricity in their homes and they don't use telephones. Their main mode of transport is still the horse and buggy and they are a very active farming community. They eat a traditional Northern European diet high in energy from protein and fat and are as obese as other Americans. However, they have about one-half the prevalence of Type 2 diabetes compared to the general population. This, scientists believe, is because physical activity, independent of body weight, seems to protect them.

> Exercise is the natural way to lower blood sugar levels and help prevent the onset of Type 2 diabetes

The risk of hypoglycemia during exercise

Because glucose is used as a source of fuel during exercise, the small levels of glycogen commonly stored in the muscles and liver can get depleted, increasing the risk of low blood sugars or hypoglycemia.

If you require insulin or a drug that stimulates your pancreas to secrete more insulin to control your diabetes, physical activity can potentially cause a low blood sugar or hypo. These include sulphonylureas (for example: Glimel™, Diamicron™, Minidiab™)

or glimepirides (for example Amaryl™) alone or in combination with an incretin (for example, Byetta™) or a dipeptidylpeptidase 4 (DPP-4) inhibitor (for example, Januvia™). Hypos are far less likely to occur if you take a biguanide (for example, Metformin™, Diabex™, Diaformin™ or Glucophage™) or a glitazone (Actos™, Avandia™). If you are on diet alone to treat your diabetes then hypos are unlikely to occur because, to prevent this from happening, the body will even break down muscle to make glucose if it has to.

> Insulin injections and certain blood sugar tablets that stimulate the pancreas to secrete more insulin increase your chances of having hypoglycemia

So if you start to experience regular hypos, then your medication may need to be reduced otherwise you will find yourself having to treat them by eating refined carbohydrate all of which defeats the purpose of doing the exercise in the first place.

> Exercise naturally reduces your requirement for insulin and blood sugar medications and these may need to be reduced to help prevent regular episodes of hypoglycemia

We used to take adolescents with Type 1 diabetes on camps in the countryside where they were given daily physical challenges like running, rowing, and abseiling and kept far more active than usual. We had to reduce their dose of insulin quite significantly when they arrived at these camps to prevent hypos. Their doses were regularly adjusted after that if they continued to experience them.

My patient from a TV reality weight-loss show was doing anything between four to six hours of exercise a day—admittedly an unrealistic and excessive regime by any standards. That exercise regime, coupled with the dramatic rate of weight loss (roughly 2.5 to 3 kilograms/5 to 7 pounds per week) resulted in him gradually reducing his insulin and eventually stopping it altogether to prevent hypos. He then had to gradually reduce his blood sugar tablets and now is on no medication at all with excellent blood sugar control.

Hypos, particularly with symptoms, should be treated with some refined sugar like glucose tablets, juice, soft drink or jellybeans perhaps followed by some slow release carbohydrate like bread or fruit.

> Hypoglycemia should be treated with some fast-acting sugar like sweetened soft drink or jellybeans and followed up with some slow release carbohydrate

2. The effect of physical activity on your blood fats

While regular physical activity has been found to have no effect on cholesterol levels, it has been consistently found to lower triglycerides even in people with Type 2 diabetes.[88] A high triglyceride level often associated with low HDL cholesterol is one of the main blood fat abnormalities in diabetes.

> Exercise has been found to have no effect on cholesterol levels in patients with Type 2 diabetes

High intensity, regular aerobic activity (pushing yourself while walking, running, swimming, rowing) is known to increase the good HDL cholesterol. However, most studies have failed to show an improvement in patients with Type 2 diabetes perhaps because of the relatively low intensity that these patients are able or willing to achieve.[97]

> Regular exercise lowers triglycerides and may raise HDL cholesterol in people with Type 2 diabetes

Unlike your car that runs on one fuel, your body can run on more than one fuel at a time. Usually when one exercises, the body burns up both sugars and fats in different proportions depending on many factors including duration of activity, level of fitness and diet. The longer the duration of the exercise the more fat is used as a source of fuel. Also the fitter one is the more fat (triglycerides) and less sugar is used up so one lasts longer. That is why fitter athletes take longer to 'hit the wall'—a term often used when the body runs out of sugar reserves in muscle and liver glycogen and the athlete feels totally drained of energy. Nevertheless, exercise, like walking, helps lower both blood sugars and blood triglycerides.

3. The effect of physical activity on your blood pressure

Naturally, if you measured your blood pressure during a walk or a run, it would be relatively high. However, that is what you would expect. This is what we call an 'acute effect' because your heart is beating faster and pumping blood through arteries at a faster rate to supply extra fuel to the exercising muscle. However, the long-term effect of regular aerobic exercise is to lower blood pressure and those who are active suffer less from this problem. Keeping blood pressure under control is important to prevent blockage of blood vessels and reduce your chances of having a heart attack or a stroke or problems with your feet. It is also important to slow down any damage the diabetes has done to your kidneys and the retina of your eyes.

> Regular exercise like walking helps keep your blood pressure under control

4. The effect of physical activity on your weight status

As explained previously, your body stores any extra food (protein, fat, carbohydrate, alcohol) that is not burnt up in the form of fat under your skin or around your waistline. This is Nature's way of saving up for a rainy day. It's an evolutionary survival mechanism and we do it very well. This enormous average reserve of energy (in males, 10 kilograms/22 pounds, 90,000 Calories, 376,560 kilojoules; in females 14 kilograms/31 pounds, 126,000 Calories, 527,184 kilojoules) in a normal weight 70 kilogram (154 pound) person is largely in the form of triglycerides. This would be much more in an overweight or obese person. When people lose weight by doing a lot of exercise, these stores of energy are slowly burnt up as a source of fuel. If we go back to our bank account analogy it is like slowly chipping away at your savings.

Studies have shown that regular physical activity alone, even without dieting, does burn up fat stored under the skin and around the waistline but may not result in overall loss in body weight as shown on the scales but in body measurements. You might find your waistline shrinking which is a very positive outcome. This is explained by the corresponding increase in body muscle with fat loss with regular exercise.[88] So, regular physical activity remains an important component of any weight management program.

A. The weight-loss phase

Normally, food restriction is more responsible for initial weight loss while regular physical activity helps more in maintaining weight loss and preventing weight regain long-term.[98] This is because an energy deficit of 500 Calories (2092 kilojoules) a day is required to lose half a kilogram (1 pound) of fat per week so it is easier to cut back on the equivalent of a meat pie than it is to walk for two hours every day. To lose one kilogram (2 pounds) a week you would have to walk four hours a day. In my experience 30 minutes a day is the most I expect of my patients and that only creates a deficit of 120 Calories (502 kilojoules) a day, nowhere near enough. There are many patients who even find 30 minutes of walking a day impossible. So it is much easier to create that deficit by cutting back on food than it is to exercise.

A friend of mine just recently bought a lawn mowing franchise for his son to help get him started in life. After one week the son decided lawn mowing was not his cup of tea. His father, a painter by trade who had invested $40,000 in the business, decided to take on lawn mowing for a while to cut his losses. In four weeks he lost five kilograms (11 pounds) and has never felt better, nor has he looked better.

As mentioned earlier, my patient from the TV reality weight-loss program had lost around 70 kilograms (154 pounds) when I first saw him. Doing four to six hours a day of exercise, and burning anything between 1500 Calories (6276 kilojoules) and 2000 Calories (8368 kilojoules) a day in the process, coupled with a reduction in energy intake, would have played a major role in his weight loss. So, in theory you can lose weight by exercising, however, most are unwilling or unable to do so due to age and other medical problems.

So, in the initial stages as one cuts back on food to lose weight, it is not unusual to experience losses of 2 kilograms (4.4 pounds) in the first two weeks, most of which is water not fat. However, this is an indication that you are eating less than your body is spending and on your way to losing weight. As the body gets used to less food, the rate of weight loss slows down. One eventually goes through short periods of two to four weeks called 'plateaus' where no loss occurs at all. This is a survival mechanism where one's metabolism drops to adjust to less food. There comes a time when hardly any weight loss occurs. At this frustrating stage, when most people are tempted to give up, exercise that increases your metabolism becomes even more important. So, if you want to get over those plateaus the best way is to exercise regularly. Get those legs working. Exercise becomes even more important after each successive plateau you go through.

> Although exercise contributes to energy deficit, cutting back on calories is easier and far more effective during the weight loss phase

B. The maintenance phase

After weight loss and during the maintenance phase, research continues to show that it is those who exercise regularly that keep the weight off.[99] That is also my observation working with overweight people over the last 25 years. Data from weight loss studies suggest that 60 to 75 minutes of moderate intensity activity like walking or 35 minutes of vigorous activity (like jogging) daily is needed to maintain this long-term weight loss.

> Exercise seems to play more of a role in maintaining weight loss

Exercisers also end up with better muscle tone, particularly if they do resistance training with weights and experience changes in body composition; they burn up fat and build more muscle.

Metabolically, muscle is a more active tissue than fat. This means the more muscle you build the higher your metabolism and the more food you can eat without gaining weight. That explains why men generally have a higher metabolism than women and can afford to eat more.

> The more muscle you build the more food you can afford to eat and get away with

Even those who do a lot of regular physical activity may not experience weight loss if they compensate for the energy they have spent by eating more. Remember, you can go and walk for an hour but you can easily make that up with one chocolate bar.

> Moderate exercise may not result in weight loss unless you watch your food intake at the same time

My patient from the reality TV weight-loss show went from 174 kilograms (383 pounds) to 104 kilograms (229 pounds) by the time I first saw him. He is aiming to get back to 93 kilograms (205 pounds) which was the healthy weight he used to be in his fighting fit days. If and when he reaches that weight, he will have to adopt a realistic exercise regime of may be an hour or so a day, and not the four to six hours he has been normally doing which is totally unrealistic. His energy intake from food would then have to be adjusted accordingly, and I would like to follow him up regularly to give him the best chance of maintaining that goal. It will be interesting to see if he can manage.

How much activity should you do a day?

Health authorities recommend 30 minutes of moderate intensity aerobic activity like walking on most, ideally all, days of the week. The American College of Sports Medicine also recommends that resistance training be included in fitness programs for adults with Type 2 diabetes.[100]

Remember those ancestors exercised several hours a day. They did that out of necessity and certainly not out of choice. We must change our attitude and think of movement as a necessity and not a choice. Is 30 minutes of walking per day really too much effort? You can make a great difference to your health by going out for that regular walk. You do not have to do it all in one go to lose weight. Your car would burn up the same amount of fuel if you drove it for three 10 minute sessions a day or only one half-hour session. It all adds up.

Similarly, your car would burn up the same amount of fuel going from point A to point B irrespective of whether you drove at 20 kilometres per hour or 40 kilometres per hour. You would just get there twice as fast. However, a recent survey[101] provides support for encouraging those with Type 2 diabetes who are already doing moderate intensity exercise to consider increased intensity exercise in order to obtain additional benefits in both aerobic fitness and blood sugar control.

The main advantage of strenuous aerobic physical activity is cardiovascular fitness. However, many of us are unable to do this for medical reasons (arthritis, heart trouble, high blood pressure). So if you can get clearance from your doctor, also enjoy some regular vigorous exercise three to four times per week to improve your cardiovascular fitness. Personally, for the benefit of aerobic fitness, I go to the gym and have a high intensity work-out on a stationary bike, treadmill or a step machine for at least 30 minutes three times per week.

> Patients with Type 2 diabetes are encouraged to do some strenuous aerobic activity for cardiovascular fitness if it is safe for them to do so

If you have not done any exercise for a while, start out by getting off that couch and changing those TV channels instead of using that remote control. Graduate to walking slowly, but regularly, and you will find that you will pick up the pace with time, as you get fitter. You will find that you cover more distance in the same time and then also get the benefits of cardiovascular fitness.

Most people think that you have to take time out to exercise but you could take advantage of your daily routine at work to increase your activity level instead. Gradually aim for 10,000 steps a day on your pedometer. Leave the car behind and walk to the shops, do not take the elevators, take the stairs. Get off the bus a block before your destination and walk the rest of the way. You will soon find yourself doing an extra half an hour a day.

> Try to exercise for 30 minutes daily to help control your diabetes. Exercise helps you lose weight by burning up body stores of fat. It also increases your body muscle-to-fat ratio and increases your cardiovascular fitness.

Does it have to be walking?

The answer to that is no. Any exercise where you use those large body muscles aerobically will do. Examples include swimming, cycling (even stationary), dancing and rowing. Combining that with resistance training using weight machines is also encouraged. There are also many varied and interesting exercise classes available for all levels of fitness: dancing, aerobics, circuit training, water aerobics, tai chi, bush walking groups, golf, bowls and 50-plus classes.

> For good results, try to combine some aerobic activity like walking with some resistance training like weights

If you do choose to walk find yourself a nice park, a beach or a shopping mall where you would enjoy walking. We know that walking is probably the best exercise for you. It is weight bearing and hence strengthens your bones, lowers blood sugars, is aerobic and hence improves your cardiovascular fitness (heart, lungs and blood vessels). It is least risky and above all it is free. I do my exercise in front of the TV. I walk for 30 to 45 minutes on the spot with dumbbells watching the news on the days I don't go to the gym.

> Finding an exercise that you enjoy is very important. If you are unable to exercise, consult an exercise physiologist for a program that you may even be able to do in the comfort of your own home.

It's so common to see older people in our Diabetes Clinic who are willing but unable to do any serious exercise. Remember that there is always an exercise that suits your needs. If you have physical or medical reasons that restrict your movements you may want to seek advice from an exercise physiologist for a safe and individually sustainable tailored program that you can even do in the comfort of your own home.

> Activity is a necessity not a choice

EXERCISE—SUMMARY
- Improves insulin sensitivity
- Reduces blood sugars
- Reduces the need for blood sugar tablets and insulin
- Reduces blood triglycerides
- May increase good HDL cholesterol
- Improves blood pressure
- Is important to lose weight and keep weight off long term

EXERCISE in a hunter/gatherer society
How much and what sort of exercise would you be doing?
- A mixture of aerobic and resistance exercise but mostly walking and running
- Many hours a day that would help you lose excess weight, lower your blood fats and blood sugars

6: The Lifestyle Factor — Food

The effective treatment of diabetes and its Metabolic Syndrome risk factors, includes not only regular activity, but a return to wholesome food habits followed by your hunter/gatherer ancestors, to food choices which adequately cover your known nutrient requirements for vitamins, minerals, antioxidants, essential amino acids, essential fatty acids, fibre[102], and to a way of eating more in harmony with Nature.

> Returning to Nature's ways will take care of all your 'Metabolic Syndrome' risk factors: blood sugars, blood fats, blood pressure and weight

Food—Nature's way

We are 'back to basics' again. Thank goodness humans have evolved to eat both plant and lean animal foods. In most cases, where both plants and animals were available it is so much easier to pluck fruit off a tree, dig for a tuber, and gather grasses than it is to catch a rabbit. So, wherever it was available, plant products constituted a major part of the diet. A scientist called Himsworth published a paper early last century showing that in different countries the more plant products people consumed as part of their staple diet, the less likely they were to get diabetes in the first place.

That is so true when you compare the incidence of obesity and diabetes in traditional third world countries where carbohydrate is the staple to that in Western countries where vegetables and unprocessed carbohydrate foods have largely been sacrificed for more refined carbohydrates, fat and protein generally.

> Eating relatively more 'plant' (particularly greens) and adequate 'animal' protein will generally help your overall diabetes control

Omnivorous humans

There is ample evidence that Paleolithic humans ate both plant and animal foods as hunter/gatherers. Whenever and wherever it was available, hunter/gatherers consumed lean animal food also.

Other animals are less fortunate and less adaptable. For example, most grazing animals like sheep and cows are strictly herbivores equipped with a special digestive system (four stomachs including one large fermentation vat called a rumen) to handle plant fibres and can only live on plant foods. Other animals, on the other hand, like the feline family are predatory and largely live on animal flesh. These are carnivores specially equipped with canines to rip flesh and a digestive system to handle a very high-protein diet.

Human beings are a bit of both and so much more adaptable. They were able to adapt to virtually all the climate zones and environmental niches on the planet, from the Arctic to temperate zones to the tropics. The human body is an amazing piece of machinery. It can actually run on four different fuels; protein, fat, carbohydrate and even alcohol for a short time if it has to.

Depending on individual tastes, availability and environmental conditions, humans in different parts of the world live on diets hugely varied in their proportions of plant to animal products, of fats, types of fats, proteins and carbohydrates. For example, Eskimos live largely on protein and fat from marine animals (mainly poly-unsaturated fish oils) and very little plant foods. However, they need this high-fat diet to generate heat to help maintain body temperature in those severe and bitterly cold conditions. Most of that fish fat is burnt up in the process of regulating body temperature. They could not survive on lettuce leaves.

On the other hand, people on the Indian continent and Asia largely live on carbohydrate and protein from plant products (grains, seeds, legumes, tubers and vegetables) with relatively small amounts of animal protein. This adaptability undoubtedly is the secret to our success as a species. In developed Western countries, however, where degenerative diseases are far more prevalent, animal products high in fats have taken over from the plant products; more meats (both fresh and processed) and certainly far more dairy products. Fats in Western countries constitute a large part of the diet (35 to 40 per cent of total calories) and unfortunately are largely the bad saturated fats that all authorities agree we should be cutting back on.

> Reducing animal fats in the diet is a message all nutrition and health authorities agree on

So, humans have evolved to be far more adaptable to combinations of foods, both of plant and animal origin. However, we should not lose sight of the fact that we have lost those long canines and have molars to help crush fibrous plant products such aas vegetables, fruits, grains and tubers.

Is the amount of food you eat important?

What seems to be of utmost importance is the amount of food one eats compared to one's level of activity. Throughout human history acquisition of food was always linked to gathering or hunting which required high-energy expenditure. I'll never forget a documentary I saw. A tribeswoman was digging out a cubic metre of soil to find one small tuber worth about 60 Calories (251 kilojoules). She must have spent many more calories doing it—Nature's way of staying lean. Typically, hunter/gatherers burnt up more energy getting food than we do today. They were always lean and remained so all their life irrespective of the proportions of animal to plant products in their diet. It is so important to achieve a realistic healthy weight for good health. My mother's uncle died at 97 years of age. I asked him once 'What's your secret to longevity and good health?' His answer was 'always get off the table hungry'.

> The single most important dietary factor that is often overlooked is the total amount of food eaten or total caloric intake

There is ample evidence in many animal species to show that restricting energy intake improves health overall and increases lifespan.

However, what is also important is variety in the diet, the balance between plant and animal foods to ensure adequate intakes of all the fifty or so nutrients that our bodies need. The proportions recommended for adult patients with obesity and diabetes is shown in a new Healthy Food Pyramid that has been evaluated and recommended by dietitians and nurses specialising in the field of diabetes education.[103] This is part of a diet kit for educators used Australia wide.[104]

Leafy green vegetables are free and strongly recommended at the expense of both carbohydrate and protein. The proportion of total calories from Carbohydrate including fruit varying between 40 to 55 per cent of total calories, Protein between 15 to 30 per cent and Fat between 25 to 30 per cent (with saturated fat plus trans fatty acids limited to 8 per cent).

> The proportions of Carbohydrate, Protein and Fat can vary in the diabetic diet depending on many factors—both physical and medical and hence the importance of individually tailored diets by a qualified dietitian

I use the well-known concept of the 'Traffic Light Guide' to help explain the diet.[105] Let's go through each of the tiers in the pyramid and see what you could change to help control your diabetes.

RED LIGHT FOODS (STOP) Tier 4

YELLOW LIGHT FOODS (SLOW DOWN) Tiers 2 and 3

GREEN LIGHT FOODS (GO) Tier 1

Healthy Food Pyramid

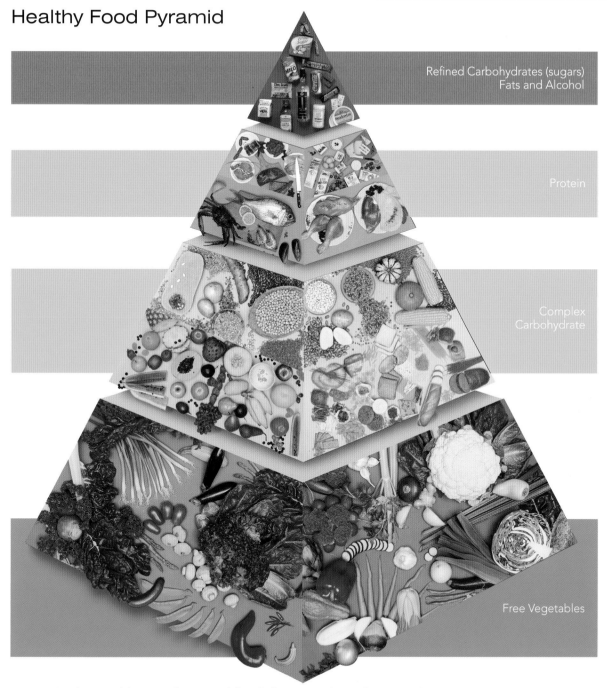

Refined Carbohydrates (sugars) Fats and Alcohol

Protein

Complex Carbohydrate

Free Vegetables

Figure 9. The Healthy Food Pyramid for diabetes and weight control

7: Green Light Foods = Go
FREE VEGETABLES

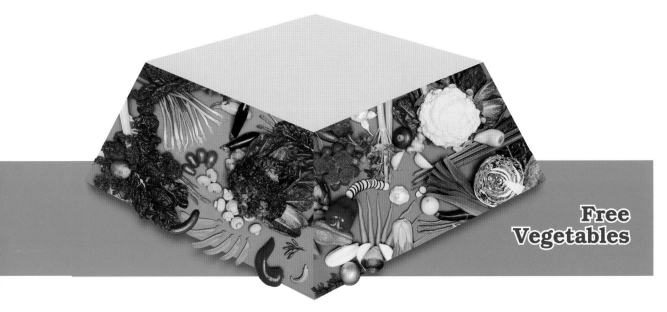

Free
Vegetables

Green light foods largely include leafy vegetables and not the starchy ones.

The effect of free vegetables on your weight

Do you know that water is the only natural food or drink that does not contain any calories and so cannot make you fat. Because leafy vegetables are around 85 to 94 per cent water, they are the next best thing—very low in calories and the least fattening of all foods. They are like those 5 cent coins that don't make much of a difference to your bank account. For this reason, many recent popular weight-loss diets are actually based on these vegetables.[106] Because they fill a gap and help control hunger, they have a major role to play in weight-loss diets and you should take advantage of them every day.

Health authorities in Australia have recently recommended five serves a day for general health, not only for weight loss but also for general health as they are rich in anti-oxidants, vitamins C, B-Carotene and fibre,[107] a target most Australians do not meet.

The higher you move up the pyramid from Tier 1 to Tier 4, the more energy dense food items become and therefore the more fattening. You would have to eat seven full lettuces to take in 500 Calories (2092 kilojoules) which would almost be physically impossible to do. However, you would only have to eat 240 grams (8 ounces) of reasonably lean steak to make up the same number of calories.

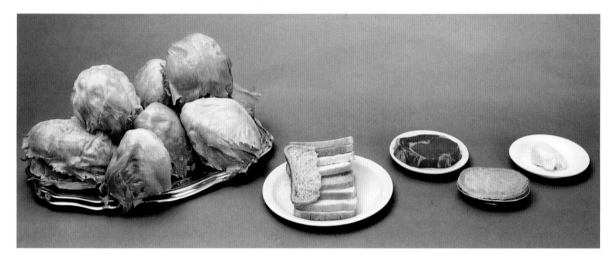

Figure 10. The energy density of foods representing the four tiers of the pyramid (each of these items contains 500 Calories–2092 kilojoules)

However, if you have a weight problem, watch the amount of fats or oil you use with vegetables as this could greatly increase your caloric intake. It is amazing how you can double your caloric intake by adding a small amount of oil in a dressing; adding four tablespoons of oil to seven lettuces doubles the Calories from 500 to 1000.

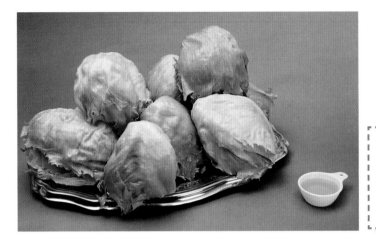

Figure 11. The effect on calories of adding oils to vegetables. Each of these items (7 lettuces and only ¼ cup/60mls/4 tablespoons of oil) contains 500 Calories (2092 kilojoules).

> Limit the oils you add to your vegetables if you have a weight problem. It is not an issue otherwise.

Health authorities combine fruits and vegetables in their health messages. However, in people with diabetes and/or a weight problem, fruits, which contain 10 to 24 per cent carbohydrate by weight, must be separated from these free vegetables that contain significantly less carbohydrate (up to 7 per cent by weight).

Since most people can not relate to calories, I will be using 'Bread Slice Equivalents' later on to illustrate the energy in foods—a concept most find much easier to understand. One 'Bread Slice Equivalent' being equal to the calories in a 30 gram slice of bread containing 70 Calories or 293 kilojoules. Example: one small apple (125 grams), one small potato (75 grams) each contains one 'Bread Slice Equivalent'.

The effect of free vegetables on your blood sugars

Leafy vegetables contain insignificant amounts (up to 7 per cent by weight) of carbohydrate, which is what ends up as sugar in your blood, and so they do not have a significant effect on your blood sugar levels. You would have to eat a whole medium size lettuce to get the carbohydrate found in one slice of bread (30g) , a small apple (125g) or a small potato (75g).

> Because of the low carbohydrate content of leafy vegetables, most people could not eat enough of them to significantly affect their blood sugar levels

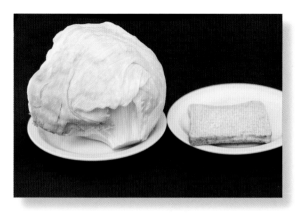

One lettuce = 1 slice of bread (30grams)

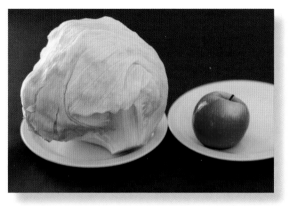

One lettuce = 1 small apple (125 grams)

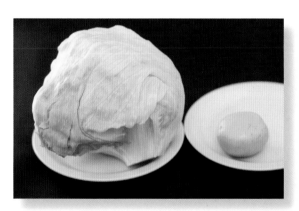

One lettuce = 1 small potato
(75 grams)

Figure 12. The insignificant amounts of carbohydrate in 'leafy vegetables' compared to carbohydrate foods

The effect of free vegetables on your blood pressure and blood fats

Green leafy vegetables can help control blood pressure in many ways. They are low in sodium salt and high in potassium. The Western diet is much too high in sodium (table salt) and low in potassium and eating more greens will help restore that balance. They also contain no cholesterol or fat, are a reasonable source of fibre and hence will help lower your cholesterol and triglyceride levels particularly when eaten at the expense of carbohydrate and protein.

Eating free vegetables at the expense of carbohydrate and protein foods can help your diabetes generally

Try to fill half of your plate with greens for your one main meal of the day.

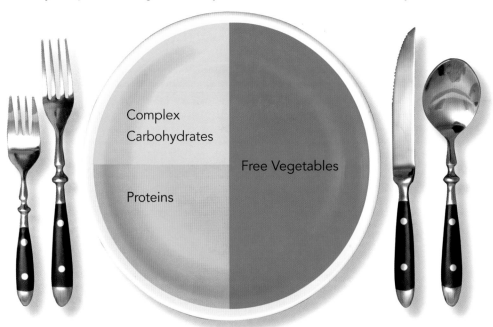

Figure 13. Recommended Plate Model: proportions of Free Vegetables, Proteins and Complex Carbohydrates on your plate

Think green, think smart and get the volume without the calories

I really think that we, as Westerners, do not eat anywhere near as much greens as our Asian, Middle Eastern and Mediterranean counterparts. A typical Western meal would be a steak covering half the plate, a couple of potatoes and two string beans.

When you are used to eating a typical Western diet with the strong tastes of fat, salt and sugar, you are unlikely to appreciate the subtle taste of greens. Once you start to cut back on fats, sugars and salt in your diet you may start appreciating their subtle taste. This is exactly what happened to my patient from the TV reality weight-loss show who lost 70 kilograms (154 pounds) and eventually controlled his diabetes on diet alone after being on both insulin and blood sugar tablets. He finally discovered the subtle taste of 'greens' after giving up on all the refined and processed takeaway foods (hamburgers, chips etc) and soft drinks. He actually loves his greens now!

You would have to have refined taste buds to appreciate the sweetness of a snow pea, mange tout/sugar pea, a string bean or broccoli. Meanwhile, to help, you might have to add a dressing to make those salads taste nice or ginger, garlic, herbs and spices.

Try my favourite salad dressing recipe for use on all salad and cooked vegetables (see page 111). You might have to make some nice soups, stir fry those greens or even make a curry to increase your vegetable intake. You might want to start your meal with a soup or salad. Fill yourself up before you start on your carbohydrates and proteins. You won't have much room for that extra bit of pasta or meat.

FREE VEGETABLES—SUMMARY
- The generous use of leafy vegetables rich in antioxidants (vitamins C, ß-Carotene) is strongly recommended
- Try to eat five serves per day as recommended by health authorities at the expense of protein and carbohydrate
- They are mostly water and the least fattening foods. They are like 5 cent coins and contribute very little to your bank account
- They contain very little carbohydrate and so hardly affect your blood sugars
- They may help reduce blood pressure and blood fats
- Try to cover 50 per cent of your plate with these vegetables
- Watch the amounts of fat and oil you use on vegetables if you are overweight

VEGETABLES in the hunter/gatherer's diet
How would you eat your vegetables, grasses and leaves?
- Most likely raw, steamed or boiled packed with Nature's goodies
- The important thing is you would not be adding any fat—sour cream, mayonnaise or oil

13 Green Light Recipes

Fresh Salads

Tabbouli Salad
Serves 6

Ingredients
1 medium Spanish onion
3 bunches parsley
1 bunch mint
4 large tomatoes
2 medium Lebanese cucumbers
4 spring onions
1/4 cup dry bulgur wheat, soaked in water for 10 minutes
2 lemons, juice and rind of one lemon
1/2 cup extra virgin olive oil
Salt and pepper, to taste

Preparation
1. Chop the Spanish onion very finely and mix well with salt and pepper.
2. Wash all vegetables and herbs and finely chop and mix with onion.
3. Add the soaked bulgur wheat to the vegetables.
4. Add the lemon juice and rind and olive oil and mix well.
5. Adjust salt and pepper to taste.

P.S. This is great with grilled meat, chicken, fish or pork.

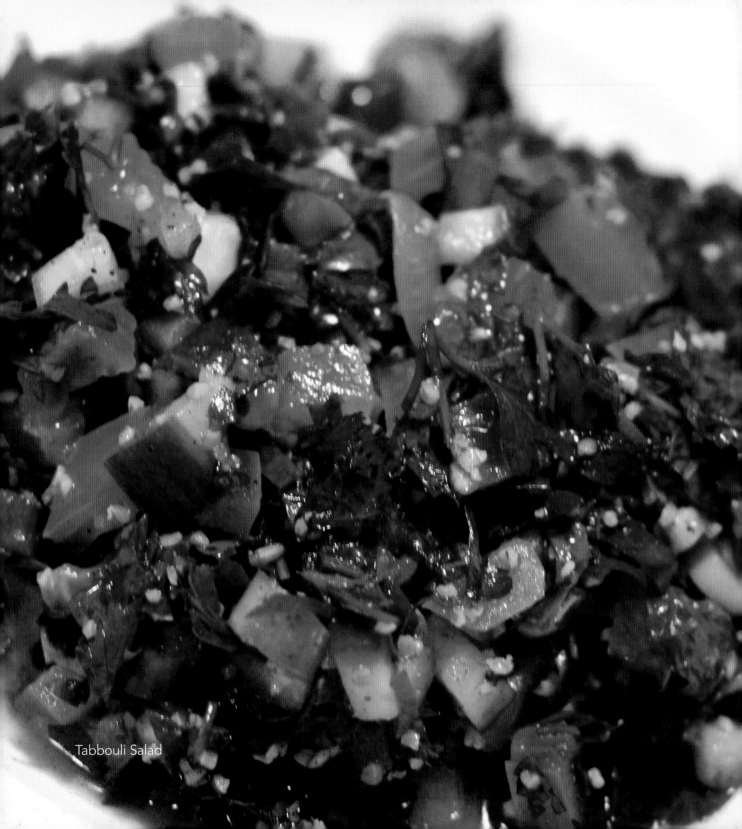
Tabbouli Salad

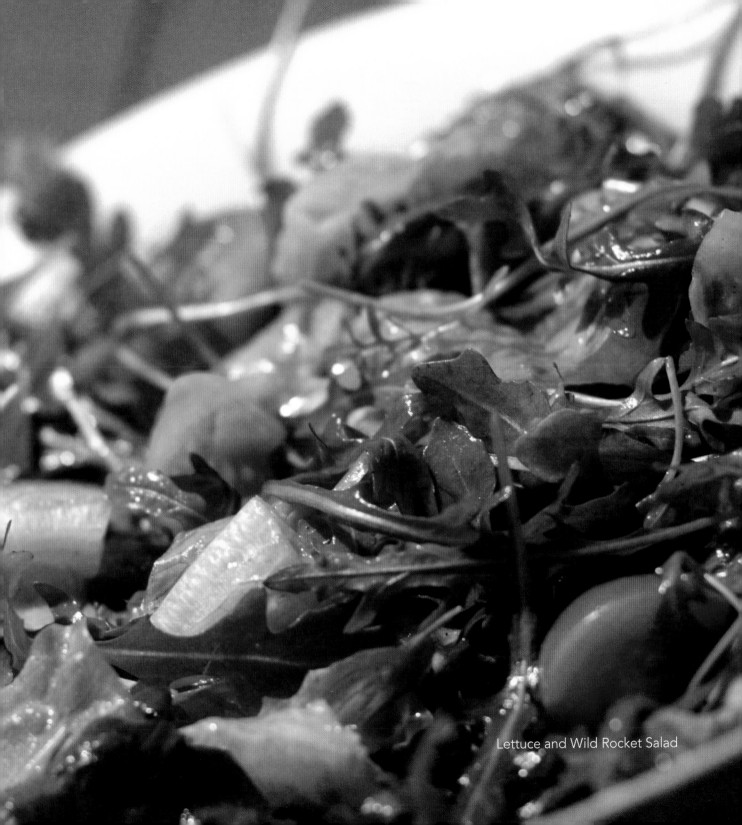
Lettuce and Wild Rocket Salad

Lettuce and Wild Rocket Salad
Serves 4

Ingredients
½ Cos lettuce
4 medium tomatoes
2 large handfuls of wild rocket
1 clove garlic
1 lemon, juiced
¼ cup white balsamic vinegar
3 tablespoons extra virgin olive oil
salt and pepper, to taste

Preparation
1. Wash all vegetables and herbs.
2. Chop the lettuce roughly.
3. Slice tomatoes into eight pieces each.
4. Crush garlic in a mortar and pestle, mix with the olive oil, lemon juice, vinegar, salt and pepper.
5. Add dressing to the vegetables and mix well.

P.S. This is nice with steak or grilled chicken. Adjust vinegar, lemon juice, salt and pepper to taste.

Fattouche Salad

Serves 6–8

Ingredients

½ lettuce

2 bunches parsley

1 bunch mint

½ medium red capsicum

3 spring onions

5 medium tomatoes

3 medium Lebanese cucumbers

1 medium Spanish onion

2 loaves Lebanese bread

½ cup extra virgin olive oil

2 tablespoons sumac

1 lemon, juiced

1 tablespoon vinegar

Salt and pepper, to taste

Preparation

1. Wash vegetables and herbs and drain dry.
2. Toast the Lebanese bread under the grill on both sides and break into 4cm (2ins) pieces in a bowl. Add the olive oil and sumac to the bread and mix well and put aside.
3. Cut lettuce into strips. Chop up parsley, mint, capsicum, spring onions, tomatoes and cucumbers. Mix vegetables together.
4. Finely chop Spanish onion. Add salt, pepper and a pinch of sumac. Mix thoroughly and add to vegetables.
5. Add the lemon juice, vinegar, a pinch of salt and pepper and mix well.
6. Just before serving, add the vegetable mix to the crunchy bread with its oil and sumac. Mix again and serve.

P.S. You can add more sumac, lemon juice, vinegar or salt to taste. Sumac is a red herb extracted from a shrub in the Mediterranean countries that has an astringent acid flavour. It is available from Middle Eastern delis. Do not forget to take into account the carbohydrate from bread. Each serve contains roughly one exchange of carbohydrate.

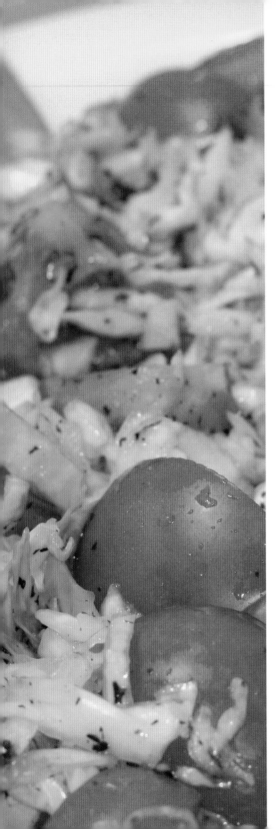

Cabbage Salad
Serves 4

Ingredients
¼ cabbage
1 tablespoon salt
4 medium tomatoes
2 cloves garlic
2 lemons, juiced
2 tablespoons extra virgin olive oil
1 teaspoon French mustard
1 tablespoon dried mint
Salt and pepper, to taste

Preparation
1. Finely chop the cabbage. Add 1 tablespoon of salt, mix very well with your fingers and leave aside to stand for 5 minutes.
2. Cut tomatoes into eight pieces each.
3. Crush the garlic in a mortar and pestle with a pinch of salt and pepper. Add lemon juice, olive oil and mustard. Mix well.
4. Wash the salt off the chopped cabbage under cold running water and drain for a few minutes. Mix cabbage in a bowl with the tomatoes, dried mint and the dressing.

PS: Adjust salt and pepper to taste.

Tomato and Cucumber Salad
Serves 4–6

Ingredients
5 medium firm tomatoes
4 medium Lebanese cucumbers
½ bunch of fresh mint
1 medium Spanish onion
⅓ cup balsamic vinegar
3 tablespoons extra virgin olive oil
1½ teaspoon of salt
1 teaspoon of black pepper

Preparation
1. Cut tomatoes into 8 pieces each.
2. Cut cucumbers into thin circular slices and add them to the tomatoes.
3. Coarsely chop mint leaves and add to vegetables.
4. Finely chop the onion and mix it well with the salt and pepper before adding it to the other ingredients.
5. Add vinegar and olive oil.
6. Mix well and serve.

P.S. Adjust pepper to taste.

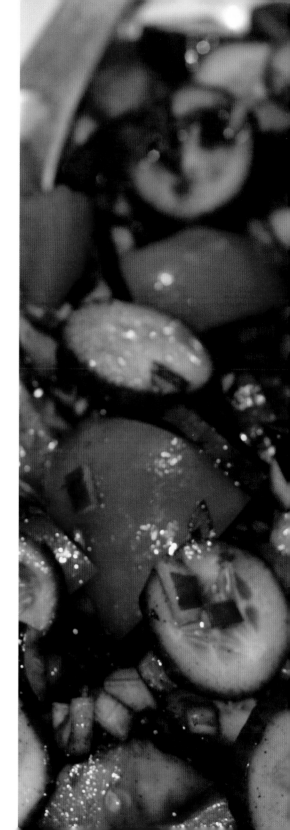

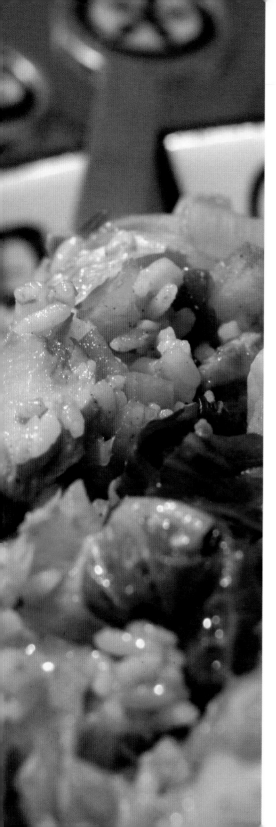

Tuna Salad
Serves 8

Ingredients

1 cup basmati or brown rice
½ medium Cos lettuce
4 medium tomatoes
½ green capsicum
½ red capsicum
1 large Spanish onion
370g (12oz) canned tuna, drained

3 tablespoons of extra virgin olive oil
3 tablespoons of balsamic vinegar
1 lemon, juiced
Salt and pepper, to taste

Preparation

1. Boil the rice until cooked. Wash with cold water and let it drain.
2. Chop lettuce, tomatoes, and capsicums and mix in a large bowl.
3. Finely chop the onion. Add salt and pepper to onion and mix well before adding to vegetables.
4. Add the rice and tuna to the vegetables and then add the olive oil.
5. Season with salt, pepper, vinegar and lemon juice. Mix well and serve fresh.

P.S. Adjust vinegar, lemon juice, salt and pepper to taste. Do not forget to take into account the carbohydrate from the rice. Each serve contains 1½ carbohydrate exchanges. This dish can be eaten as a meal as it contains protein, carbohydrate and vegetables.

Tomato Salad
Serves 4-6

Ingredients
6 medium tomatoes
1 large Spanish onion
1 lemon, juiced and rind grated
1 tablespoon white balsamic vinegar
3 tablespoons of extra virgin olive oil
Salt 1½ teaspoons
Pepper 1 teaspoon

Preparation
1. Chop tomatoes into 8 pieces each.
2. Finely chop onion and mix it well with the salt and pepper then add to tomatoes.
3. Stir in lemon rind.
4. Pour over the lemon juice and vinegar.
5. Add olive oil and mix well.

P.S. Adjust salt, pepper, lemon and vinegar to taste. Enjoy with grilled fish.

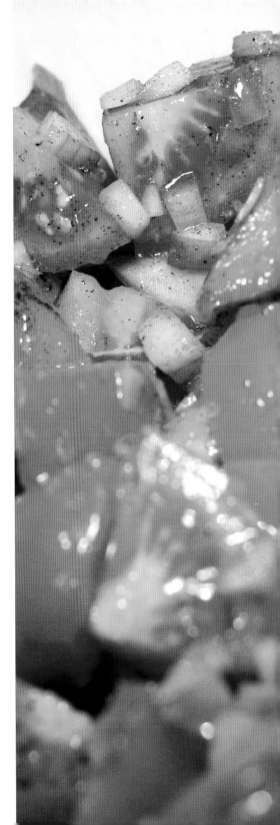

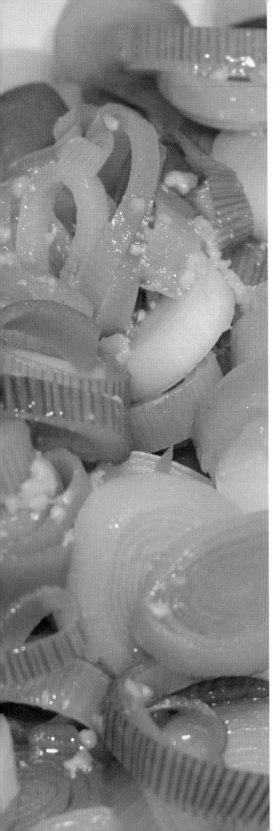

Steamed Vegetables

Leeks Vinaigrette

Ingredients:
3 leeks
Vinaigrette dressing (see recipe opposite)
Salt and pepper, to taste

Preparation
1. Boil water in a steamer.
2. Use the white part of the leeks only.
3. Wash leeks thoroughly after cutting them length-wise into 5cm (2in) pieces if small and 1cm across if large.
4. Steam for around 10 minutes or until soft.
5. Cool under cold water or in a bowl and drain well.
6. Arrange on an hors d'oeuvre dish.
7. Add dressing.
8. Serve hot or cold.
9. Adjust salt and pepper to taste.

Other vegetables that lend themselves well to the same steaming process:
Bok choy, broccoli, cabbage, cauliflower, asparagus, snow peas (mange tout), string beans, artichokes and Brussels sprouts. Most of these, other than Brussels sprouts and artichokes, will take far less time to cook than the leek. These can be served as an entrée or as an accompaniment to your main meal. They can be eaten cold.

Vinaigrette Dressing

Ingredients
4 tablespoons balsamic vinegar
1 clove fresh garlic
2 tablespoons extra virgin olive oil
1 teaspoon French Dijon mustard
A pinch of salt and pepper

Preparation
1. Finely chop the garlic and crush in a mortar and pestle with a touch of salt to make a paste.
2. Add the olive oil, balsamic vinegar and mustard and mix thoroughly.

You might want to use some lime or lemon juice with or instead of the vinegar for variety. White balsamic vinegar could also be used for presentation instead of dark vinegar.
If you are concerned about your weight, reduce the olive oil even further.
If you do not have a weight problem, then for better balance and taste, you could reverse the ratios of olive oil and balsamic vinegar.

8: Yellow Light Foods = Slow Down
CARBOHYDRATES

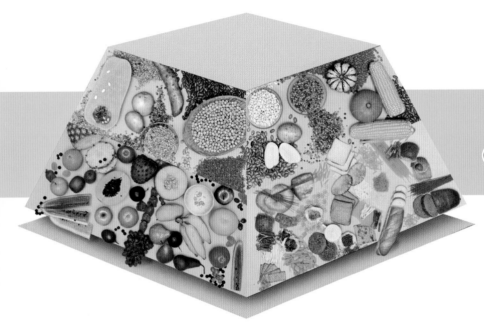

Complex Carbohydrates

All plant products other than green leafy vegetables are carbohydrate foods. These include both **starches** (found in grain products, starchy vegetables and legumes) and **simple sugars** (like fructose, glucose and sucrose found in fruits).

> Carbohydrate is found in plant foods mainly fruits, grains, starchy vegetables and legumes

Chemically, sugars and starches are classified according to the number of sugar units in their structure. Simple sugars are either monosaccharide, containing only one sugar molecule (for example glucose, fructose, galactose) or disaccharides containing two sugar molecules linked together (for example sucrose, commonly known as table sugar, lactose, the sugar in milk and maltose commonly known as malt). Starches on the other hand, are polysaccharides containing many glucose molecules linked together in a straight (amylose) or branched (amylopectin) chain. Many other polysaccharides exist in nature but most can't be digested by humans and are classified as non-starch polysaccharides or dietary fibre that the body does not absorb.

1. The effect of carbohydrates on your blood sugars

Carbohydrate is an important source of energy in the human diet. Different sources of starch (carbohydrate) are used in the diet depending on where you are in the world. In Far East Asia rice and noodles are the main staple. In the Middle East it is bread. On the Indian subcontinent breads, rice and legumes remain the staple foods. In Africa, the staple varies from banana to millet to wheat depending on availability. In the Pacific Islands, vegetables like taro, tapioca, sweet potato, yams, and fruits like unripe banana and breadfruit are used as a main source of carbohydrate. In Western countries potato and bread have been main sources of carbohydrate, however, with the influx of migrants from all over the world this is slowly changing.

What has to be remembered is that all carbohydrates (both simple sugars and starches) are ultimately absorbed, and converted in the blood stream to a sugar called glucose. So when you measure your blood sugars with a glucometer you are in fact measuring the glucose concentration in your blood.

> Both simple sugars and starches are ultimately converted to the sugar called glucose in the blood

Glucose is a vital source of energy for all body tissues, especially the brain, and for that reason, the body tries to maintain a constant level of glucose in the blood at all times (between 4.0 and 8.0 mmol/l). In normal circumstances, when blood glucose levels rise after a meal of carbohydrate, surplus glucose is removed with the help of insulin and taken up by body cells to give you energy thus restoring blood sugar levels to normal in the process. Any excess is ultimately and inefficiently converted to fat and stored away. On the other hand, after prolonged fasting, before a meal or while exercising, a minimum level of glucose in the blood is maintained by breakdown of a stored sugar called glycogen (in muscle and liver).

Are fruits included in the carbohydrates?

Yes. Fruits are included in with the carbohydrate foods like bread and potato. A common recommendation by health authorities is to 'eat plenty of fruit and vegetables'. That may well be the case for general health but when you have diabetes and/or a weight problem; you have to think of fruit as a carbohydrate that needs to be somewhat restricted. Keep in mind that a large apple and a medium banana each contain the carbohydrate equivalent of two slices of bread. A couple of serves of fruit a day is adequate.

How are sugars made in nature?

Sugars are made by plants only—a process called photosynthesis. Plants take in carbon dioxide from the air through special holes in the leaves called stomata and mix it with water taken in by the roots in the presence of sunlight (energy) to make the sugar glucose (see Figure 14). Many glucose molecules linked together make starch.

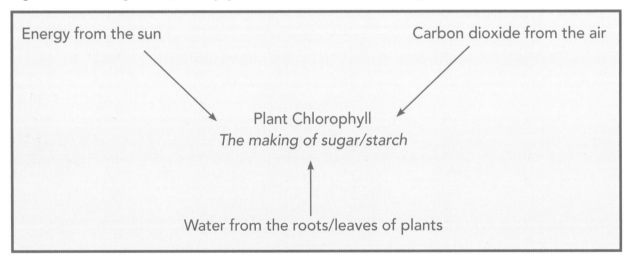

Figure 14. How plants make sugar (glucose) and starch

Only plants are capable of this process because it is in the chloroplasts, in the leaves, that contain the green substance chlorophyll, that this process takes place. There is no sugar in unprocessed animal products like hard cheese, egg, meat, chicken, fish, pork, veal and seafood. There is, however, only one unprocessed animal product that does contain sugar, and that is milk for obvious reasons. Baby animals are not capable of chewing plant foods and rely on milk only for their source of sugar so nature provides.

> There is no sugar in unprocessed animal products like hard cheese, egg, meat, chicken, fish, pork, veal and seafood

These plant products are different to leafy vegetables in the sense they contain mainly carbohydrate that eventually ends up as sugar in the blood stream. One can understand why fruits end up as sugar because they are sweet. However, most people have difficulty believing that bland starchy foods like bread, potato, rice or pasta that are not sweet, also eventually end up as sugar in the blood. All you have to do to prove that is check your blood sugars one hour after eating a plate of rice, or pasta or some bread. You will soon realise that they end up as sugar too.

Why do starchy foods end up as sugar in the blood even though they are not sweet?

Well, the answer lies in the make-up of starch. Starch is in fact made up of many sugar molecules called glucose linked together like beads in a rosary. When they are linked in a straight chain, the starch is called amylose and when they are linked in a branched form, the starch is called amylopectin. When a starchy food like bread is eaten, it gets partially broken down by the process of chewing with saliva in the mouth and completely digested in the small intestine by enzymes to individual glucose molecules. Only then are they absorbed into the blood stream. It's like breaking down a rosary into its individual beads. Remember, starch as is, can't be absorbed and has to be broken down into its glucose components for the body to use it.

You have to start thinking of starchy foods like breads, rice, pasta, potato and corn as sources of sugar even though they are not sweet

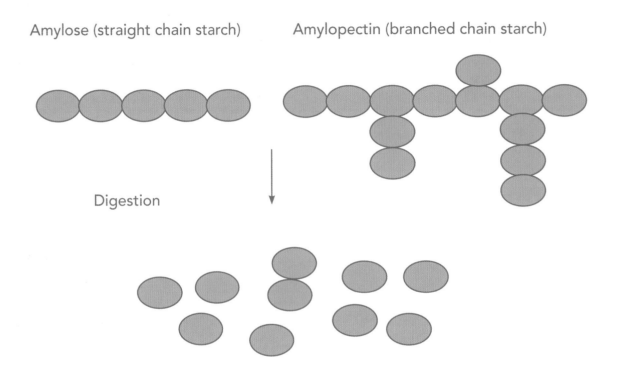

Amylose (straight chain starch)   Amylopectin (branched chain starch)

Digestion

Individual glucose molecules (which are then absorbed into the bloodstream)

Figure 16. The digestion of starch (Amylose and Amylopectin)

Steps you can take with carbohydrates in your diet to help control blood sugars

Both the quantity and type of carbohydrate determine the Glycemic Load of a meal (GL) and hence blood glucose and insulin levels after eating. The total amount of carbohydrate consumed is the strongest predictor of how high your sugars are going to go.[108] However, selecting the right type of carbohydrate (those with a low GI, Glycemic Index) is very important.[109]

> Both the amount and source of carbohydrate determine the 'Glycemic Load' of a food or a meal

STEP 1. Limit the quantity of carbohydrate in your diet

If someone has diabetes, carbohydrates should not be eaten in quantity at any one time. After all, diabetes by definition is an intolerance to carbohydrate and so it's common sense to reduce the Glycemic Load (GL) of a meal. Not only do carbohydrates end up as sugar but also any excess that is not burnt up is stored away as fat. They are like those $20 notes, take enough of them to the bank and you will soon find they make a difference to your bank balance. That is why carbohydrates belong to The Yellow Light foods—slow down.

> All carbohydrate foods end up as sugar in the blood stream and for that reason their intake must be somewhat compromised to help your blood sugars and your weight

Gone are the days of large plates of rice for Far East Asians and pasta for Italians with diabetes and a weight problem. Gone are the days of plates of legumes on rice eaten with bread for Middle Easterners with diabetes. That does not mean that people with diabetes can't eat carbohydrates but they have to compromise their intake. Try to restrict carbohydrates to a quarter of the plate.

STEP 2. Space your carbohydrate evenly over the day

Carbohydrates must be spaced out over the day. It's like putting 20 litres of petrol in your tank three times a day as apposed to putting 60 litres in all at once. Small and often is the way with carbohydrate.

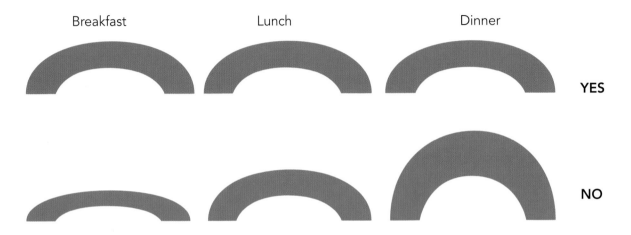

Figure 17. Recommended carbohydrate spacing over the day

Carbohydrate foods should be spaced out over the day

By doing so you are not straining your pancreas to produce extra insulin. By the same token, it is also important to have some carbohydrate and be consistent with the amounts at each meal, to balance the effect of blood sugar tablet and or insulin you may be taking. See Meal Plans later in the book for a typical menu showing the even distribution of carbohydrate over the day.

STEP 3. Choose the low-Glycemic Index (GI) carbohydrates

For the best sugar results and to reduce the Glycemic Load (GL) of a meal it is most important to reduce the amount of carbohydrate at each meal, and also to select the best carbohydrate foods—the low-GI foods, those that are known to raise your blood sugars least.

For the best part of this century, the most widely held belief, even among nutritionists and dietitians, was that simple sugars like table sugar needed to be avoided and replaced by so-called complex carbohydrates or starches, for example, bread and potato. This was based on the false assumption that simple sugars are more rapidly digested and absorbed into the blood stream than starches and hence would raise your blood sugars to a greater extent. This has proven to be largely wrong since the concept of the Glycemic Index (GI) was introduced in 1981 by a Canadian researcher called David Jenkins as a more accurate method of assessing and classifying peoples' blood sugar response to carbohydrate containing foods.[110]

The GI is a relative ranking expressed as a percentage of carbohydrate containing foods according to their effect on blood glucose levels when fed to people and compared to a standard. As a result of these studies carbohydrate foods are now classified into Low (equal to or less than 55 per cent), Medium (between 56 and 69 per cent) or High (equal to or greater than 70 per cent) GI foods. Obviously, the lower the GI the less it raises your blood sugars.

Table 11. The Glycemic Index rating

Low GI	55 or less	(Recommended)
Medium GI	56–69	
High GI	70 or more	(Not recommended)

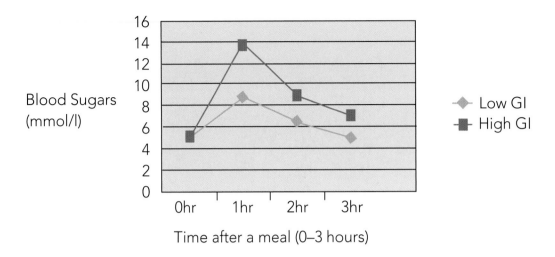

Figure 17. Comparing the effects on blood sugars of the same amount of carbohydrate from a 'high' and a 'low' GI food

Hundreds of foods have been studied to date and their GI values are available from the University of Sydney at their website www.glycemicindex.com or best-sellers put out by Australian researchers.[111, 112]

As of June 2002, in Australia, many food products containing carbohydrate have been labeled with the Glycemic Index tested logo. This is now a simple way to shop for healthy low-GI choices. To have this logo, products must have had their GI tested at an approved testing facility and meet strict nutrient criteria for calories (kilojoules), saturated fat, dietary fibre and in some cases calcium, to ensure they are all-round healthy choices. To find out more about the GI-tested logo visit www.gisymbol.com.

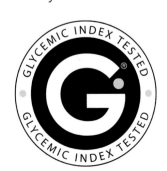

Figure 18. The GI-tested logo applicable to carbohydrate foods

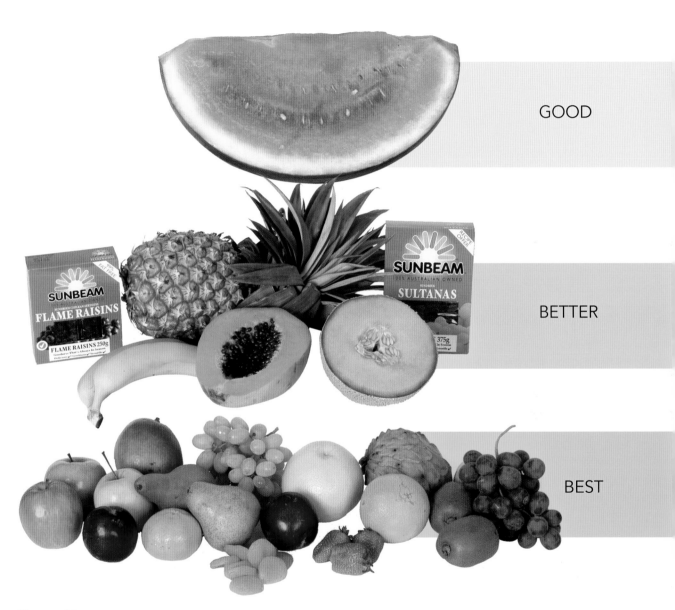

GOOD

BETTER

BEST

Figure 19a. The GI of fruits

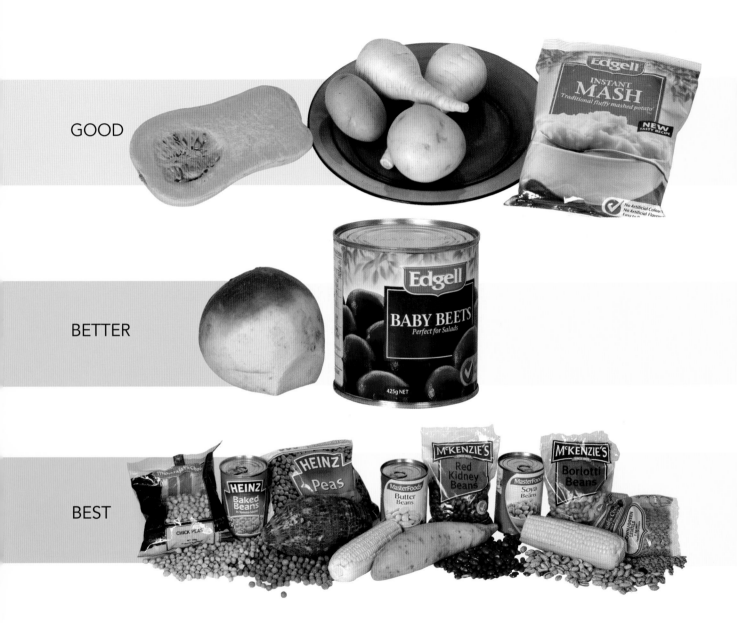

GOOD

BETTER

BEST

Figure 19b. The GI of starchy vegetables

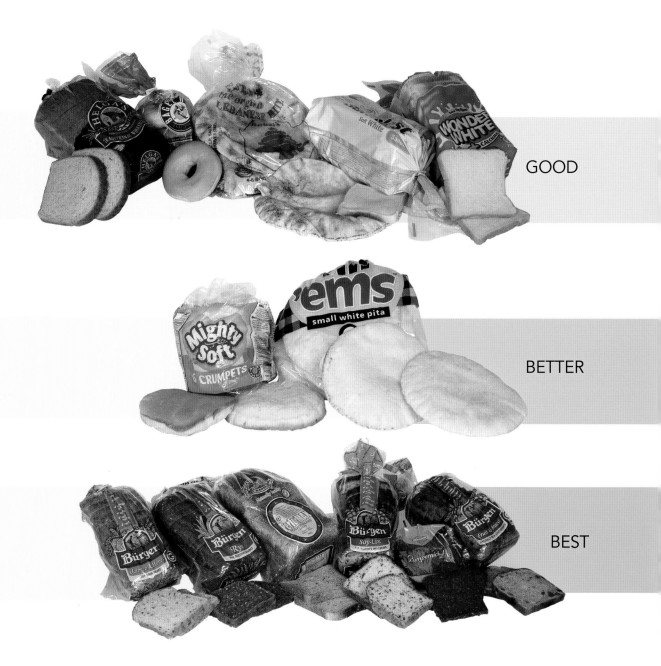

GOOD

BETTER

BEST

Figure 19c. The GI of breads

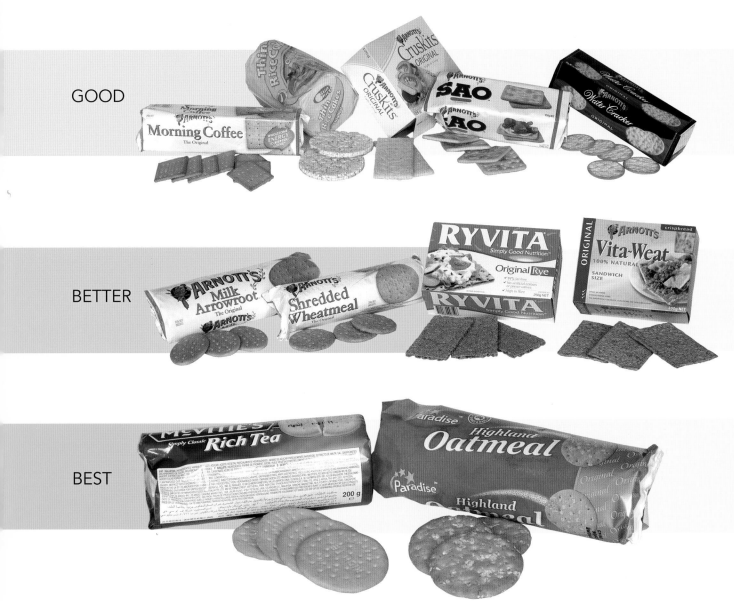

GOOD

BETTER

BEST

Figure 19d. The GI of Biscuits

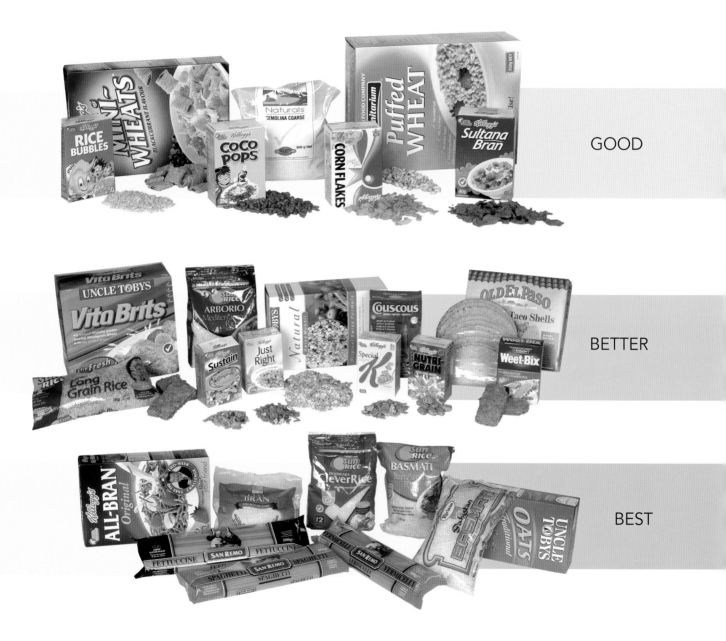

Figure 19e. The GI of cereal foods

What determines the GI of a carbohydrate food?

There is a direct relationship between the rate a carbohydrate food is digested, the rate it raises blood sugars and the amount of insulin required to restore normal blood sugar levels. The slower the food is chewed, digested and absorbed, the less it raises blood sugars and the lower its GI. As a general rule, the less processed the food, the less it raises your blood sugar and the less insulin is required. As expected, traditional, unrefined, unprocessed bush foods eaten by our hunter/gatherer ancestors mostly have low GIs.[113]

> The more processed or refined a product the faster it will be digested and the higher it will raise your blood sugars

Some factors that affect the rate of digestion of a carbohydrate food and hence its GI include:

1. **The form of the carbohydrate food.** Multigrain breads that need to be chewed and digested slower have a lower GI than white or even wholemeal breads that have fibre, but have been processed by milling.

> Multigrain breads are better than white or whole meal for blood sugar

2. **Raw versus cooked carbohydrate foods.** Generally, cooking carbohydrate foods speeds up the process of digestion and results in higher blood sugars. The best example is a raw potato that cannot even be digested at all. Cooking a potato, however, ruptures the starch vacuoles and releases the starch making it easy to digest. Similarly, stewing an apple would result in higher sugars than eating the fresh apple for obvious reasons.

> Generally, the less cooked a carbohydrate food is, the less it raises your sugars

3. **The type of starch in the food.** There are two types of starch: one which is a straight chain of glucose molecules called amylose and another branched chain called amylopectin which is easier to break down and digest. Certain types of rice are amylose-rich and are recommended because of their relatively low GI.

> Carbohydrate foods containing mostly amylose starch are harder to digest and hence have a lower GI

4. **The type of sugar.** As mentioned earlier, there are many types of naturally occurring sugars. One sugar called fructose, mainly found in fruits and therefore commonly known as 'fruit sugar' raises blood sugars much less than glucose because it is not all converted to glucose in the blood. It has a low GI of only 23. Because of their fructose content, fruits generally raise blood sugars less than dry savoury biscuits (which are mainly starch or glucose). For that reason, it is preferable to eat fruit and not biscuits for snacks.

> Temperate climate fruits like citrus fruits (orange, mandarin, grapefruit etc), stone fruits (peaches, plums, apricots, cherries, nectarines etc), berries (strawberries), apples and pears raise blood sugars less than tropical fruits and melons

5. **The presence of fat in the food.** Generally, the presence of fat in a food would lower its GI because fat slows down the rate of stomach emptying and hence digestion. However, even though a lot of fatty foods may have a low GI (chocolate has a GI of 49; ice-cream, 61; potato crisps, 54; shortbread biscuits, 48), one should not choose these regularly if they are trying to lose weight or have elevated blood fats.

> Those with a weight and/or cholesterol problem can only afford to eat low-GI foods that are high in fat sparingly

6. **Acidity in foods.** Acid in foods slows down the process of digestion and results in a lower GI. Citrus fruits containing citric acid have a very low GI partly for that reason. That is probably why grapes have a lower GI compared to raisins.

> The use of vinegar (acetic acid) or lemon juice (citric acid) in food preparations (for example, salad dressings) is recommended to lower GI

7. **The presence of soluble fibre.** Soluble fibre mainly found in oats and barley slows down their rate of digestion. The way oats and barley go gluggy when cooked is what helps slow their digestion and absorption. Try to include oats in breakfast cereal, oat-bran biscuits and barley and oat-based breads in your diet.

> Cereal products (breads, biscuits, breakfast cereals) based on oats and barley have the lowest GI and are recommended in preference to wheat products to lower blood sugars

8. **Legumes also commonly known as pulses** such as lentils, kidney beans, butter beans, soybeans, peas and chickpeas have been around and used for centuries in South America, Far East Asia and the Middle East. However, their use in Western countries has generally been very limited. They have a very low GI and help control blood sugars and blood fats.

Table 12. Factors that determine the GI of a carbohydrate food
• The form of the food (refining of grain products like bread)   • Raw versus cooked starches (potato)   • The type of starch (amylose versus amylopectin)   • The type of sugar (glucose versus fructose)   • The presence of fat in foods (ice cream)   • Acidity in food (raisins versus grapes)   • The presence of soluble fibre (barley, oats)

STEP 4. Include at least one low-GI food with every meal

It is advised that people with diabetes include at least one low-GI carbohydrate food per meal if not all. An example of that would be oats (porridge) for breakfast, multi-grain bread for lunch and lentils, Basmati rice, pasta, sweet potato or corn for dinner.

> It is not enough to limit the quantity and evenly space carbohydrate over the day. You should preferably select low-GI carbohydrates to lower Glycemic Load (GL) and blood sugars after meals.

STEP 5. Watch the quantity of low-GI foods

One of the most common mistakes for people following a low-GI diet is the false sense of security they fall into with excess carbohydrate being eaten only to find their weight not moving and their sugars not improving. Remember, even if it is a low-GI carbohydrate, you will not get away with eating too much of it. I have seen so many patients who have even sacrificed green vegetables and protein to eat more low-GI carbohydrate, in the belief that it is better for them, only to find their waistline expanding, their sugar control deteriorating and their need for diabetic drugs increasing.

> Even if the carbohydrate you are eating is of low GI, you will not get away with eating too much of it: your sugars will not improve and you may not lose any of that extra weight

How do you calculate the Glycemic Loal (GL) of a carbohydrate food?

Do not forget that both the GI of the carbohydrate food and more importantly, the amount consumed, determine the Glycemic Load (GL) of that food and the extent to which that food will raise your blood sugars. Carbohydrate serves are classified as 'low GL, less than 10'; 'medium GL, 10 to 20' or 'high GL, 20 or more' (see Table 13).

Table 13. The Glycemic Load (GL) rating	
Low GL	10 or less (Recommended)
Medium GL	10–20
High GL	> 20 (Not recommended)

Let's calculate the GL of an apple as an example. A small apple (125 grams) contains 15 grams of carbohydrate and has a GI of 38. It has a GL of

GL = GI (38) x 15 (amount of carbohydrate in that serve) /100 = 5.7 (Low)

What about a small baked potato containing 15 grams of carbohydrate with a GI of 85?

GL = GI (85) x 15/100 = 12.7 (Medium)

So we would expect the baked potato to raise your blood sugars more than twice as much as the apple.

How do you calculate the Glycemic Load (GL) of a carbohydrate meal?

The GL of a meal can be calculated from the GL of individual carbohydrate foods in that meal. If you ate both the apple and the baked potato together then the GL of that meal would be 5.7 + 12.7 = 18.4 (medium GL). So the GL of a meal is much more predictive of the effect this meal would have on blood sugars than the amount of carbohydrate or GI alone (see Figure 20).

The higher the GL of the meal or snack the higher the blood sugars will be and the more insulin will be required to restore normal blood sugars. Furthermore, eating too much of a low-GI carbohydrate could raise your blood sugars even more than eating small serves of a high-GI carbohydrate.

Figure 20. The effects of 'low' and 'high' Glycemic Load (GL) meals on blood sugars over the day

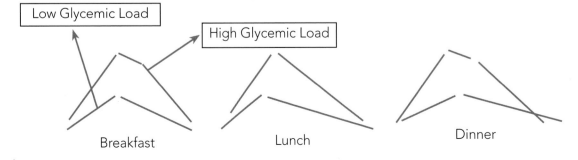

How can you reduce the Glycemic Load (GL) of your meals?
 » Reduce the amount of carbohydrate at your meals and increase protein and free vegetables instead
 » Choose low-GI carbohydrates instead of high-GI carbohydrates (for example, multigrain bread instead of white bread)
 » Choose smaller amounts of the medium to high-GI carbohydrates (white breads, potato, jasmine rice, watermelon)

> The most effective way to lower the Glycemic Load is to choose low GI foods and limit their portion sizes

Can you have any Moderate to High-GI carbohydrates?
Of course, but if you want to keep your Glycemic Load (GL) low you should only have these in small amounts to compensate for the high GI. Perhaps these can be eaten as a treat or for snacks. For example, watermelon has a high GI of 72. But if you only have one cup which contains only 8 grams of carbohydrate, the GL equals = 72 x 8/100 = 6 which is a low GL. Even if you had two cups it would make it a medium GL of 12.

Why are fresh fruits generally better than juices?
Our hunter/gatherer ancestors ate fresh berries and other fruits as Nature provided. They certainly did not drink juices. Hunter/gatherers had no choice of drinks, it was water or nothing. What a different world we live in today. Every year hundreds of new beverages including fruit juices come onto the market to target our innate fondness for anything sweet.

   The difference between fruit and juices is that when you juice a fruit you remove all the fibre that normally slows down digestion and you are concentrating the calories. By refining fruit that way you can drink much more than you can eat, significantly increasing both your sugar (GL) and caloric intake.

   Have you tried eating three oranges in one sitting? No. But you can easily find yourself drinking their equivalent in sugar on a hot day. Each time you drink half a cup of juice you are eating the equivalent of an orange (15 grams of carbohydrate and 70 Calories, 293 kilojoules or 1 'Bread Slice Equivalent'). Next time you line up at that

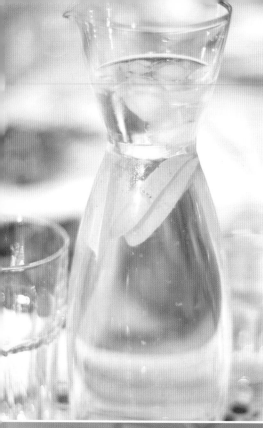

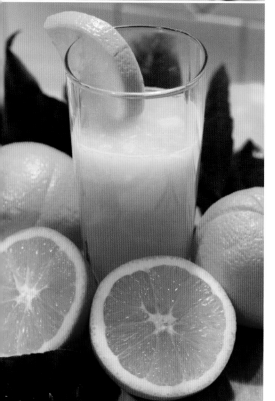

fruit juice counter, just take a note of how much fruit is used to make your juice.

What if the fruit juice was natural with no added sugar?

Well, do not be deceived by this marketing ploy. It does not really make much difference because there is only 2 per cent difference in the sugar content of fresh juices (8 per cent sugar) and sugar added juices (10 per cent sugar). They don't really need to add much to natural juices, as they are already very sweet. Another reason not to drink juices is the fact that fructose (fruit sugar) in quantity may raise triglycerides—a blood fat abnormality already present in many people with Type 2 diabetes.

What is the best way to eat your grain products?

How did your ancestors eat the grains they gathered? They certainly did not send them to the mill and do what we do. We get rid of all the fibre (bran) in the seed, all the vitamins in the aleurone layer and end up with this white fluff called 'starch' and if we're lucky, get some added back by the manufacturers. Research has shown this added fibre does not work in the same way and hence does not have the same health benefits. Gatherers may have partly ground their seeds but it re-mained largely rough with all the fibre and vitamins in the flour. These rough products are generally chewed slower, digested slower and hence absorbed into the blood stream slower. That is why multigrain breads and multigrain biscuits have a lower GI than either their white or wholemeal counterparts.

STEP 6. Consult your Accredited Practising Dietitian (APD) for the amounts of carbohydrate to eat at each meal

The amount of carbohydrate prescribed is determined by many factors including your age, sex, weight status, blood sugar status, normal carbohydrate intake and your level of activity. Diabetic associations recommend around 50 to 55 per cent of total calories should come from carbohydrates. However, this has been challenged somewhat by recent research (the CSIRO Wellbeing Diet and others) that shows that reducing carbohydrate to 40 per cent and substituting more lean protein (30 per cent instead of 15 per cent) in the diet can also help with weight loss and reduce blood fats.[83, 84] The long-term effects of these relatively higher protein levels on kidney function in people with diabetes remain to be seen.

   The dietitian may describe a set of Carbohydrate Exchanges for each meal and snack. A Carbohydrate Exchange is described as the amount of carbohydrate food containing 15 grams of carbohydrate. See Table 18, page 181, for a short list of Carbohydrate Exchanges of low-GI foods. For a more comprehensive list of Carbohydrate Exchanges, see The Traffic Light Guide to Food, 2005'[105] which can be purchased from Diabetes Australia.

> The amounts of carbohydrate to have for each meal and/or snack are generally determined by an individual consult with your Accredited Practising Dietitian (APD) who specialises in diabetes. Look one up in the Yellow Pages or on your Dietitians Association website

Should you have carbohydrate snacks between meals?

Well, the answer depends on many factors particularly your blood sugar status and the type of medication, if any, that you are on to lower your sugars.

   If you are on diet alone: If you are on no diabetic tablets you need not have snacks between meals.

If you are on diabetic tablets:

- » If you are on diabetic tablets that boost the pancreas to produce more insulin like Sulphonylureas (Diamicron™, Diamicron MR™, Glimel™, Minidiab™) or a Glimepiride (Amaryl™) these can cause low blood sugars or 'hypos' and snacks between meals may be indicated.
- » If you are on tablets called Biguanides (Metformin™, Diaformin™, Glucophage™ or Diabex™) or a Glitazone (Actos™, Avandia™) that reduce insulin resistance rather than stimulate the pancreas to produce more insulin, hypos are unlikely to occur and you most likely do not need snacks between meals.

If you are on insulin: There is always a risk of having a hypo when on insulin and you should be prepared to treat it with some high-GI foods.

- » If you are on two injections a day (usually a combination of a fast and an intermediate acting insulin like NovoMix™ 30, Mixtard™ 30/70 or Humulin™ 30/70), you run the risk of hypos particularly in between meals. In this case a snack may be necessary.
- » If you are on three fast acting injections (one before each meal like NovoRapid™, Humalog™ or Actrapid™) and intermediate or long acting insulin like Protaphane™, Levemir™, or Lantus™, you are less likely to have hypos.

Nevertheless, there is no guarantee and all patients on insulin should be prepared for the unexpected at any time by always carrying foods like 'glucose tablets', jellybeans or barley sugar.

Remember, where being overweight is an issue, it is always best, where possible, to lower the dose of your medication than to increase food to prevent hypos. Without exception this should be done with your doctor's or diabetes educator's consent.

> Where overweight is an issue, it is best to lower the dose of your medication in consult with your doctor, than to increase food to prevent hypos

2. The effect of carbohydrates on your blood fats

As mentioned in Part 1, the most common blood fat abnormality in people with Type 2 diabetes is high triglycerides and low HDL cholesterol as part of their Metabolic Syndrome profile. These abnormalities are associated with insulin resistance and high blood sugar levels. The first and most important measure to reverse this is to normalise your blood sugar levels initially by diet, exercise and weight loss and failing that with the introduction of sugar lowering tablets. Reducing the glycemic load (GL) by reducing the amount of carbohydrate in your diet, spacing it over the day and focusing on low-GI carbohydrate foods is the first step towards achieving this.

3. The effect of carbohydrates on your weight

In countries where carbohydrate is the staple obesity is generally not an issue. Asians eat rice for breakfast lunch and dinner yet you hardly ever see an overweight person. So it does not necessarily mean that high-carbohydrate diets will inevitably result in you becoming overweight or obese. In fact, it is in Westernised countries, where carbohydrate (rice, potato, bread) has been sacrificed for more protein (meat, chicken etc) and fat in the diet that weight seems to become a problem.

   However, carbohydrate foods are potentially fattening. They are like those $20 notes. Deposit enough of those in your account and they will certainly add up. Any excess carbohydrate you eat over and above what you require is converted to triglycerides and stored away for a rainy day. That is why you may have to compromise with these not only to help your blood sugars, but equally importantly to help you control your weight. Focusing on unprocessed, unrefined, low-GI carbohydrates has been found to help with weight loss as these carbohydrates are more filling than others, take longer to digest and so help delay hunger pangs. Choosing oats for breakfast instead of cornflakes, multigrain bread for lunch instead of white bread, Basmati rice for dinner instead of Jasmine rice and fruit for snacks instead of biscuits are just some examples.

CARBOHYDRATES—SUMMARY

- Carbohydrates are found in plants: Grains, Fruits, Starchy vegetables and Legumes
- Should be somewhat restricted if you have diabetes to reduce Glycemic Load and/or a weight problem to reduce caloric intake. Remember they are like $20 notes—take enough of those to the bank and it will make a difference
- Should be evenly and consistently spaced over the day to help control blood sugars
- Emphasis should be on low GI unprocessed unrefined carbohydrates low in fat to help reduce Glycemic Load
- See a dietitian for recommended amounts called 'exchanges' of carbohydrate—if blood sugar control remains unsatisfactory, blood fats remain high or you are failing to lose those extra kilos

CARBOHYDRATES in a hunter/gatherer's diet

How did they eat their carbohydrate foods?

- In their natural, unprocessed, unrefined, low-GI form
- With very little fat if any as no concentrated forms existed like margarine, butter and oils

9: Yellow Light Foods = Slow Down
PROTEINS

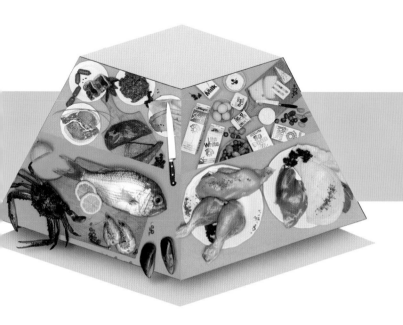

Proteins

What are the sources of protein in your diet?

The major sources of protein in the Western diet are animal products. These in the Australian diet include meat, poultry and fish (about 33 per cent) and dairy foods (about 16 per cent), cereals and cereal-based foods (about 25 per cent), and vegetables (about 8 per cent) also contribute.[114, 102] Proteins are found in both animal and plant foods and are made up of building blocks called amino acids. Understandably, the amino acid composition of animal protein is close to that found in human muscle. However, the essential amino acids, those required by our body, can also be provided in the amounts needed by adults from plant sources.

Prior to the Agricultural Revolution and the start of animal husbandry 10,000 years ago, humans would have derived most of their protein from wild animals.[34] Whatever they hunted was likely to be very lean; you can always count the ribs of wild animals. Compare a wild duck to a domesticated duck, a wild buffalo to a domesticated cow or a battery chicken that reaches slaughter weight in no more than seven weeks to its free range relative that could take up to six months to one year to reach that target. There is a big difference in the amount of storage fat.

> Humans have evolved to eat very lean meats

The effect of protein foods on your weight

Animal foods consist largely of water with an average of 65 per cent (range: 50 to 80 per cent). They also contain protein and fat in different proportions and an insignificant amount of carbohydrate in the form of glycogen. So the caloric content of a piece of meat, chicken, or fish would be determined by its protein (4 Calories or 16.7 kilojoules per gram) and fat (9 Calories or 37.6 kilojoules per gram) content. Generally, the lean proteins that our hunter/gatherer ancestors ate would have been relatively low in energy, which helped keep their weight down. However, even when protein foods are lean, they can still contribute to your weight if eaten in significant amounts. A reasonably lean 240 gram (eight ounce) steak is equivalent to seven small potatoes or seven 'Bread Slice Equivalents' in energy and is very easily consumed compared to larger amounts of carbohydrate foods.

One of the most common misconceptions I encounter in my practice is the belief that fish is not fattening. Patients often cut back on red meat and eat fish in quantities, only to find that they do not lose any weight. Remember, even white fish, lean as it may be, is protein just like lean red meat and both are potentially fattening if eaten in excess. Remember, protein foods are like those $50 notes. You do not have to take many of those to the bank to make a difference to your bank balance. Yet again, try and eat more greens at the expense of some of your protein foods. You will soon find your reserves drying up.

The effect of protein foods on your blood fat levels

The small amounts of fat on wild game consumed by your hunter/gatherer ancestors would have been structural (good poly and monounsaturated) and not storage (bad saturated) fat.[115] This would have helped significantly, not only in reducing their caloric intake, but also in lowering their risk of cardiovascular disease.

So in the wild, it did not matter whether the meat was red from a ruminant herbivore (buffalo, zebra) or white (fowl, fish and seafood) because it was mostly very lean anyway. It was a pure source of protein with very low levels of fat. Compare that to some of the high-fat meats we eat today and the many other dairy products like milks, yogurts, ice creams, butter and cream, all of which contain a lot of that nasty saturated fat. It is not surprising that a large proportion of the Western population today has a cholesterol problem. Importantly, people with diabetes have a higher incidence of heart disease and for that reason should try even harder to keep cholesterol levels within the normal range.

In adopting Western dietary habits, many ethnic groups tend to seek out and consume plenty of this animal protein and fat, something rarely done in their own countries of origin. It is a matter of availability and affordability. That may partly explain why this group, having changed its eating habits, has an even higher rate of these diseases.

We need to eat lean sources of protein just like our ancestors. The Meat and Livestock Industry has responded to consumer demands for lean cuts of meat. They have done this by open pasture, or free range animal husbandry, by feeding stock certain diets, slaughtering livestock at an early age and by removing fat at the retail level. It is up to you, the consumer, to select these lean cuts.

> Select very lean sources of protein: fish and other seafood, beef, trim lamb, chicken breasts and new fashion pork

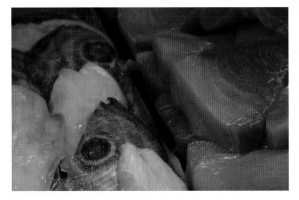

What about fish?

Fish is an excellent source of protein and can also be rich in omega 3 fish oils. White fish is very low in oils (2 to 3 per cent by weight) compared to fatty fish like mackerel, herring, sardines, trout, tuna, salmon and eels which contain anything between 11 to 18 per cent. However, these are largely polyunsaturated omega 3 fish oils: (Docosahexaenoic acid DHA and Eicosapentaenoic acid EPA [116] which may have cardiovascular health benefits for patients with diabetes. They can lower triglycerides reducing the risk of cardiovascular disease.[117] They keep platelets from getting too sticky thus decreasing the chance of having clots. From EPA your body makes PG3 prostaglandins which also help prevent cardiovascular complications accompanying diabetes.

It is recommended that people with diabetes eat fish
a couple of times a week

What about dairy products?

In Western countries we continue to eat dairy products throughout our adult lives yet in nature all animals are discouraged from suckling after they have been weaned onto solids. It would have been impossible for humans to consume milk prior to the Agricultural Revolution 10,000 years ago when livestock was first domesticated. So, on an evolutionary scale, dairy products are relative newcomers to the human diet.

It does not surprise me that 70 per cent of the world adult population is intolerant to lactose (the sugar in milk). Lactose intolerance is the inability to digest lactose causing gastrointestinal upsets, bloat, flatus and sometimes diarrhoea. It varies greatly among different ethnic groups and is highest among Asians such as Thai, Japanese, and Chinese (90 to 97 per cent) and Africans (Bantu 50 per cent; African Americans 70 to 75 per cent) where dairy products have never been a part of their ancestors' diet.

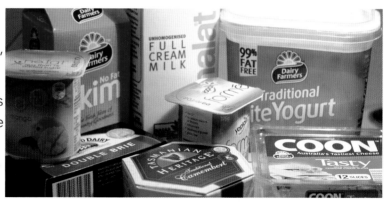

Even among Westerners it is estimated that 10 per cent are lactose intolerant. Maybe nature did not intend us to have milk as adults. I am not lactose intolerant and eat a fair amount of dairy products to get the benefits of their high calcium content. However, I make sure I reduce saturated fat by choosing low or skim milk products. Remember, in Western countries, saturated fat is the most significant contributor to our cholesterol and heart problems. For those with lactose intolerance, and depending on the degree of intolerance, small amounts of fermented dairy products and lactose-free milk or soymilk would possibly be a suitable alternative.

> Select low-fat or even skim milk dairy products like skim milk, skim milk yogurts, cottage and ricotta cheese and 97 per cent fat free cheeses if you have a weight and/or cholesterol problem

How much protein do adults need?

The answer to that is not much. You must remember that you have lost those long canines. During the growth period and throughout adolescence, you require good quality protein to ensure optimum growth potential to lay down muscle on a growing skeleton. However, when you stop growing in height, that is generally mid-teens in young females and late teens in males, you only need protein for maintenance. Any growth from then on is either outwards or downwards as that is when weight problems set in and the law of gravity starts to take over.

Only small to moderate amounts of protein are needed in adult humans because the body constantly recycles muscle (protein). All we really need is to replace essential losses or endogenous losses of protein which is lost in falling hair, shed skin and in the stool when we go to the toilet.

Adults need no more than 0.75 grams per kilogram of body weight per day obtained from both plant and animal foods (120–200 grams/4–7 ounces per day) to replace these losses. This corresponds to 10 to 20 per cent of total calories in the diet.

It is also best to spread this protein over at least two meals a day, maybe some on a sandwich at your light meal and the rest should cover no more than a quarter of the plate for your main meal of the day. Remember, no one needs two main meals per day unless they are very physically active.

When protein is added to a carbohydrate meal it is known to reduce its GI because it slows down the process of digestion—another reason to spread protein over the day. It can also stimulate the pancreas to produce insulin to help the body use sugar as a primary fuel.

> Adults need no more than 120 to 200 grams (4 to 7 ounces) of lean animal foods a day. Protein allowance is best spread over at least two meals to help lower the GI of carbohydrates

Recently there has been renewed interest in diets that are slightly lower in carbohydrate and slightly higher in lean protein that may prove to be an option for patients with diabetes that do not have any sign of kidney complications. There is no harm having a bit more protein at the expense of carbohydrate as long as it is lean and as long as you are not gaining weight. However, if there is a kidney problem related to diabetes (nephropathy) increasing protein in the diet is not advised.[78, 79, 80]

Our ancestors surely had ample protein in the diet depending on availability. Hunter/gatherers not only had lean meats but cooking it on the fire would get rid of any fat and that's how you should cook your meats too.

> Cook your meats in such a way as to reduce the fat content

What if you are a vegan (strict vegetarian)?

A vegan is someone who eats no animal products at all. As an adult, generally it is not a disadvantage to be a strict vegan as far as meeting your protein requirements. This is because one can still get adequate balanced protein from a combination of cereals and legumes. However, this can be a disadvantage for someone diagnosed with diabetes because vegan food would normally come from plant products, most of which contain carbohydrate. Perhaps including some Texturized Vegetable Protein (TVP) products and tofu in the diet could help.

PROTEINS—SUMMARY
- You do not need anymore than 120 to 200 grams (4 to 7 ounces) per day of protein foods
- Protein generally should not cover more than 25 per cent of your plate
- You could have up to 30 per cent of calories in the diet from lean protein if you have no signs of kidney damage
- Make sure that the protein you eat is lean
- Select skim or low-fat dairy products particularly if you have a weight or cholesterol problem
- Spread your protein over lunch and dinner if possible to help your blood sugars
- Select more white meat than red
- Eat fish at least twice per week

PROTEINS in a hunter/gatherer's diet
How would you be eating your meats?
- Lean because wild animals carry little, if any, extra stored body fat
- You would cook your meats on the fire so that any fat was lost in the process
- It was distributed among people in your tribe and hence consumed in small/moderate amounts. Remember that adults do not need protein in quantity

10: Red Light Foods = Stop
SUGARS

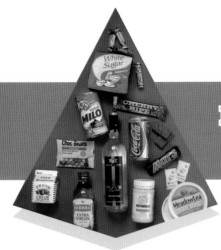

Refined Carbohydrates (sugars)
Fats and Alcohol

The red light foods include all the foods that your ancestors did not eat at all because they were not available so obviously our bodies have not evolved to eat them in quantity. Look at how much fat and sugar and alcohol we consume today. People with diabetes who are concerned about blood sugars, blood fats, blood pressure and their weight must seriously limit these foods to treats. Let's look at each of these foods individually.

Sugars

The earliest evidence of refined crystal sugar being produced dates back to 500 BC in northern India. Before this time, wild honey would have been the only concentrated form of refined sugar that humans had access to, and that would have been seasonal. Fresh fruits and berries would have been the main regular source of sugar. So our cravings for sweet foods today are a legacy of our ancient ancestors who sought these foods because they were so rare. On an evolutionary scale refined sugar is a very recent addition to the human diet.

Western countries like the US, England and Australia have consumed a large amount of refined sugar since the beginning of the Industrial Revolution 250 years ago when sugar was first produced on a commercial scale. The apparent annual sugar consumption in Australia has remained very high (up to 50 kilograms/110 pounds per person) for the last three decades with an increase in sugar consumed in manufactured foods. There has been some decrease in sugar consumed in confectionery, bakeries and as refined sugar. The greatest increase in sugar intake has been through non-alcoholic beverages like tea, coffee, soft drinks, cordials and juices.[114]

> Refined sugar has only been produced on a commercial scale and consumed in quantity by humans since the industrial revolution 250 years ago

Even though there is no strong evidence to show that sugars cause diabetes, high intakes do put extra strain on the pancreas to produce more insulin, exacerbating the underlying problem in those with diabetes or at risk of developing the disease. There is no doubt that patients who have a sweet tooth and drink two to three cans of soft drink a day (containing the equivalent of 16 to 27 teaspoons of sugar) and eat a lot of sweets benefit immensely simply by reducing or even cutting these foods out altogether. My patient from the TV reality weight-loss show used to drink nothing but soft drinks (one to two litres per meal) and now has finally discovered water. He even likes it!

What changes can you make?
Step 1. Reduce sweet foods generally
These include sugars, jams, honey, treacle, syrups, molasses, lollies, chocolates, chocolate spreads, health food bars, carob, cakes, sweet biscuits, flavoured milks, ice creams, ice blocks, soft drinks, flavoured mineral waters, tonic water, cordials, canned fruit in syrup, sweet pies and pastries.

Figure 21. The sugar in soft drinks

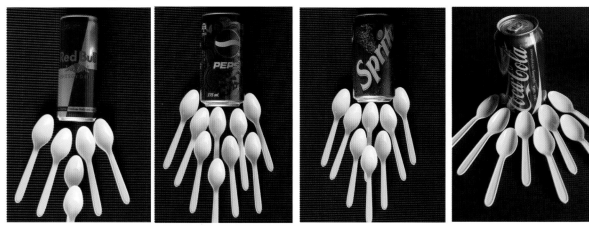

Figure 22. The sugar in Coke® versus Diet Coke® & Coca Cola Zero®

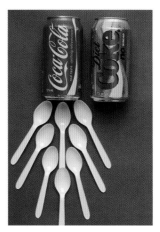 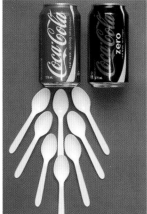

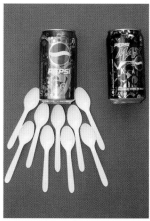

Figure 23. The sugar in Pepsi® versus Pepsi Max®

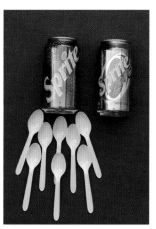

Figure 24. The sugar in Sprite® versus Sprite Zero®

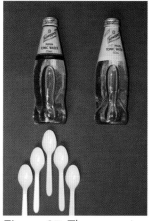

Figure 25. The sugar in Schweppes Indian Tonic Water® versus Diet Tonic Water

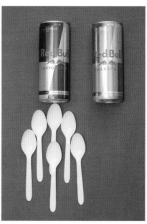

Figure 26. The sugar in Red Bull® power drink versus Red Bull Sugar Free®

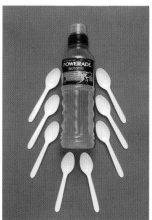

Figure 27. The sugar in Powerade® (Wallabies Gold Rush and Berry Ice)

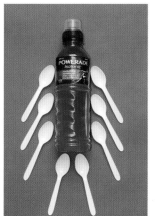

Figure 28. The sugar in 'no added sugar' fruit juice (250ml)

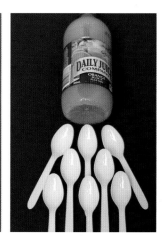

Figure 29. The sugar in 'no added sugar' fruit juice (500ml)

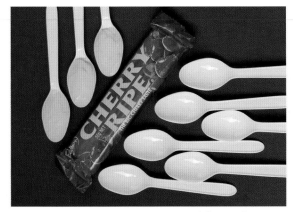

Figure 30. The sugar (white) and fat (yellow) in a Cadbury Cherry Ripe® (55 grams)

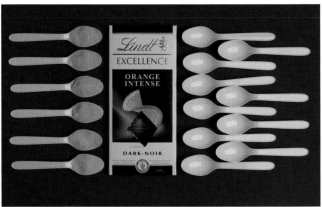

Figure 31. The sugar (white) and fat (yellow) in Lindt Orange Intense Dark chocolate bar (100 grams)

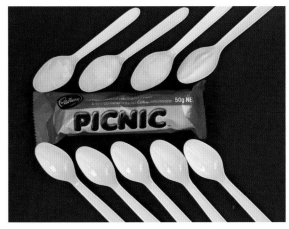

Figure 32. The sugar (white) and fat (yellow) in Cadbury Picnic™ chocolate bar (50 grams)

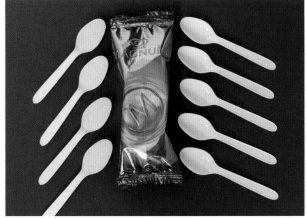

Figure 33. The sugar (white) and fat (yellow) in ice cream (Magnum Classic®)

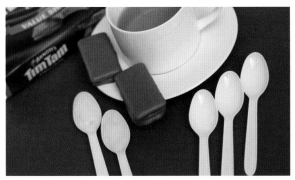

Figure 34. The sugar (white) and fat (yellow) in Tim Tam™ biscuits

Step 2. Look for low-sugar alternatives

There are alternatives that you can have that do not affect your blood sugars but solve that craving for something sweet. There are a number of alternatively sweetened products on the market that a person with diabetes can have without compromising their blood sugar levels (see Table 14). These are considered safe by health authorities.

> There are a number of artificially sweetened products on the market suitable for people with diabetes

However, there is still one disadvantage to drinking or eating these artificially sweetened foods in quantities even if they do not affect your blood sugars. As long as you are bombarding your taste buds with these sweet products, you will forever have that craving and you are more likely to attack that cake trolley when it comes around at morning tea time. If you can, in the long-term, try to use them less often as this will reduce your threshold for sweets and that piece of fruit might eventually taste sweet enough. You might even enjoy fresh water. Try and filter the chlorine from your tap water with a simple filter. Freshen it with a dash of fresh lime or lemon.

Step 3. Watch the high-fat sweets

Refined sugary products can also be high in fat. Although a lot of high-fat sweets (ice-cream, flavoured milks etc) have a low GI and do not overly raise blood sugars, fats of all kinds contain the highest number of calories. So if you feel like something sweet your first choice should be a diet or alternatively sweetened product. Your second choice could be a bit of jam or honey on toast. Your last choice, particularly if you are watching that waistline, is foods high not only in sugar but also in fat as well. There is a big difference between eating a teaspoon of jam or honey on a slice of bread and a chocolate bar that could contain three to four times the calories.

> The occasional treat of the real thing is also fine if your blood sugars are well controlled and weight is not an issue

Do people with diabetes have to cut sugar out completely?

No. It is not only the refined sugary products that end up as sugar in your blood stream. We now know that all carbohydrate foods do. We also know that some simple sugars do not raise your blood sugars any more than most starches do. In fact the GI of simple sugars (table sugar or sucrose GI=65, fructose GI=23) are lower than those so-called complex starchy foods (potatoes GI=88, Weetbix GI=70, white and wholemeal bread GI=70) that contain no sugar at all. However, be careful not to over consume these foods.

Table 14. Artificial sweeteners and products suitable for diabetes

Soft drinks:
Any diet or low-calorie/joule soft drink (Diet Coke, Coke Zero, Pepsi Max)
Low-calorie/joule tonic water
Low-calorie/joule ginger ale
Low-calorie/joule cordials

Artificial sweeteners:
Tablets: Sweetex, Sugarella, Sucaryl, Saccharin, Sugarine, Equal, Hermesetas, Splenda, Balance
Liquids: Sugarine
Powders: Equal, Splenda, Sugarless, Nutrasweet

Replacing some starch in the diet with small amounts of simple sugars should not raise your blood sugars any further. For that reason, Diabetic Associations around the world are allowing for some sugar in the diet as long as it is consistent with good blood sugar control. Some jam or honey on your toast for breakfast or a teaspoon of sugar in a couple of cups of tea or coffee a day, should really not make much difference.

There is no scientific justification for advice that people with diabetes should completely avoid all simple sugars and sugar-containing foods. This really is unnecessary.

Replacing carbohydrate in the diet with small amounts of sugar should not raise your blood sugars any further. There is no need to cut sugar out completely.

However, too much sugar in your diet cannot only raise your blood sugar levels but can take the place of healthy nutritious foods

REFINED SUGARS—SUMMARY
- Reduce sweet foods generally
- Eat sweets occasionally as treats
- Look for low-sugar alternatives
- Watch the high-fat sweets
- Do not be so concerned with small amounts of sugar in your diet as long as your blood sugars are well controlled

SUGAR in the hunter/gatherer's diet
- Very little indeed was consumed
- This indicates that humans do not need sugary foods to survive
- Sugars were largely consumed in the form of natural wild fruits and berries
- Treats were occasionally taken in the form of honey

11: Red Light Foods = Stop
FATS and OILS

It is important to note from the outset that your hunter/gatherer ancestors would certainly have eaten far less fat than you do today. This is understandable, when you consider they had no concentrated sources of fats at all like butter, margarine and refined oils.

More importantly, their animal fat intake would have been low too because wild animals are generally very lean with very little, if any, storage fat. They would have eaten moderate amounts of vegetable oils in their natural, unprocessed, unrefined form from seeds and nuts which would ensure they got the minimum requirement for essential fatty acids (linoleic acid, LA and alpha Linolenic Acid, ALA) that our body can not make and hence are required in the diet for good health.

> Our hunter/gatherer ancestors ate oils and fats in their natural, unprocessed, unrefined form

> We now know, what Mother Nature always intended, that humans do not need much oil anyway and we certainly do not need much animal fat in our diet

In Western countries, we just take in too much fats and oils. They make up a high of 35 to 40 per cent of all the calories we eat in spite of health messages to reduce fat and a food industry that has provided a plethora of low and reduced fat products. In a gatherer/hunter society this could be as low as 10 to 20 per cent and in a hunter/gatherer society as high as 28 to 39 per cent but low to moderate in saturated fats.[32]

What are fats and oils made up of?

Fats and oils in your food, as well as the fat you store on your body, are mainly made up of what we call triglycerides (more than 95 per cent). So the margarine you have on your bread, the lump of fat you eat off your steak, the vegetable oil you cook with or the oils hidden in the nuts, seeds or avocado you eat, are all mainly made up of triglycerides.

> Fats and oils in your diet are mainly made up of triglycerides irrespective of whether it is of plant or animal origin

Each triglyceride molecule, as the name suggests, is made up largely of three fatty acids that vary in their length and degree of saturation and this is what gives fats and oils their characteristics: solid fats versus liquid oils for example.

What is the difference between oils (plant) and fats (animal origin)?

We have all heard of polyunsaturated, monounsaturated and saturated fat. The number of double bonds in the chemical structure of a fatty acid determines its degree of saturation, the more double bonds the more unsaturated.

Nature arranges double bonds in these nutritionally important unsaturated fatty acids in the 'cis' form where both hydrogen atoms in the double bond are on the same side of the molecule. During processing and refining of oils, these can be converted to 'unnatural trans fatty acids' which act like saturated fatty acids because their shape has been changed. They are increasingly being used in the fast food and snack industries.

> Unsaturated oils are found in nature in their 'cis' form and not in the 'trans' form we find today in processed, refined and hydrogenated fats

Polyunsaturated oils. Fatty acids with more than two double bonds are known as polyunsaturated. They are liquid at room temperature and commonly found in most vegetable oils like corn, sesame, sunflower and safflower oil. It is recommended that polyunsaturated oils constitute around 10 per cent of total calories in the diet.

> Polyunsaturated oils are liquid at room temperature and recommended to constitute around 10 per cent of total calories in the diet

Monounsaturated oils. Fatty acids with only one double bond are known as mono-unsaturated. They are commonly found in some vegetable oils like olive, canola and peanut oil. It is recommended that monounsaturated oils constitute approximately 10 per cent of total calories in the diet.

> Monounsaturated oils are good oils, liquid at room temperature and recommended to constitute around 10 per cent of total calories in the diet

Saturated Fats. Fatty acids with no double bonds in their structure are known as saturated and are generally hard at room temperature and commonly found in animal fats like meat fats and dairy fats like butter. The two exceptions are coconut oil and palm oil as they are plant oils that are high in saturated fat. Saturated fats should constitute no more than 8 per cent of total calories in the diet.

> Saturated fats are the bad hard fats at room temperature and should constitute no more than 8 per cent of total calories in the diet

One must remember that there is no such thing as a natural fat or oil that is purely monounsaturated, polyunsaturated or saturated, they are all a mixture and it is the proportion of these three types of fatty acids that determines the degree of saturation in the final product. For example, olive oil is made up of 74 per cent monounsaturated fatty acids (the rest is polyunsaturated and saturated) and therefore is considered monounsaturated oil. On the other hand, butter is made up largely of saturated fatty acids (the rest is polyunsaturated and monounsaturated) and is accordingly known as a saturated fat.

Table 15. Types of fats/oils and where they are found

Type of fat	Where is it found?	Comments
Saturated fat *Eat least*	• Meat fats particularly from animals that chew their cud (beef and lamb) • Dairy fats from animals that chew their cud (like milk, yogurt, cream, sour cream, ice cream, butter, ghee) • Foods made with these animal fats like pastries, takeaway foods etc • Coconut and palm oil (Exceptions to most plant oils)	These fats raise your cholesterol level
Monounsaturated fats/oils *Eat sparingly in place of saturated fats*	• Extra virgin olive oil, olives • Avocado • Canola oil • Peanuts	Replacing saturated fats in the diet with small-moderate amounts of olive oil/canola helps reduce cholesterol without affecting blood sugars
Polyunsaturated fats/oils *Eat sparingly in place of saturated fats*	• Safflower oil • Sunflower oil • Corn oil • Soybean oil • Cottonseed oil • Polyunsaturated margarines • Fish oils	Replacing saturated fat in the diet with small amounts of polyunsaturated oils can help lower cholesterol levels

Unfortunately, a lot of the fat we take in today is saturated, particularly from rumi-nant animals. It is also from refined vegetable oils that have been processed from seeds: extracted with solvents, subjected to heat in excess of 150 degrees Centi-grade, degummed, bleached and deodorized thus removing a lot of the healthy natural goodness found in the seed in the process. Many of these refined oils are fur-ther subjected to the process of 'partial hydrogenation' changing the composition of polyunsaturated fatty acids from their 'natural cis' form to the 'unnatural trans' form.

This 'high saturated fat' and 'trans fat' in our diet has significant nutritional impli-cations. It increases your chances of having large blood vessel disease when you, as a person with diabetes are already at higher risk of developing cardiovascular complications.

The effect of fats/oils on your weight

As far as we know all fats and oils are equally fattening. In fact, they are the most fat-tening of all foods. They are the other extreme to water—the only substance that you ingest that contains no calories. If we go back to our bank account analogy, fats/oils are the $100 notes. You do not need to deposit many of those to increase your bank balance.

> All fats and oils are equally fattening and the most fattening of all foods

There is twice as much energy in a gram of fat (9 Calories, 37.6 kilojoules per gram) than there is in a gram of carbohydrate (4 Calories, 16.7 kilojoules per gram) or pro-tein (4 Calories, 16.7 kilojoules per gram). So if you are concerned about your waist-line, you need to focus on cutting back on fatty foods and all fats and oils irrespective of where they come from. Your body does not distinguish between the types of fat when it comes to your waistline. It is a common misconception among patients that so called healthy fats and oils are less fattening.

How to cut back on your total fat intake

Here are seven easy steps to cut back on fats found in some commonly eaten foods. The amount of fat is represented in teaspoons.

Step 1: Try not to fry but grill, microwave, steam or dry fry

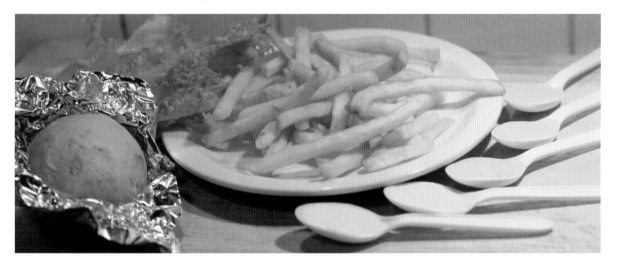

Steamed potato (130 grams) versus McDonald's large serving of fries (130 grams)

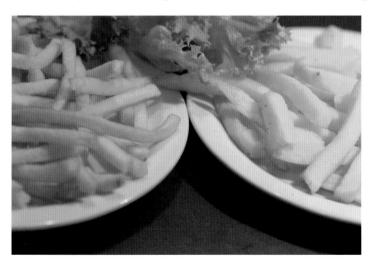

And if you have a choice always choose large fries over small fries as the latter absorb much more fat because of increased surface area.

Step 2. Trim the fat off your meats

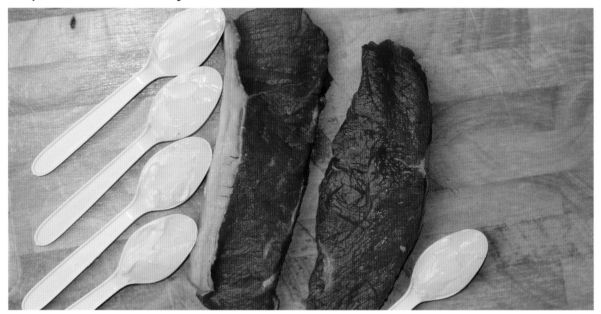

Step 3. Avoid fatty takeaway foods.

McValue meal 46 grams fat (9 teaspoons)
KFC meal   60 grams fat (12 teaspoons)

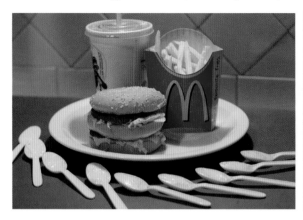
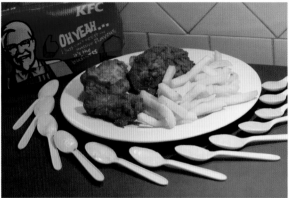

Step 4. Try low-fat or even skim milk dairy products.

1. Cheese slices (2 slices = 42 grams)

Tasty	Light & Tasty	Bega So Extra Light
14 grams fat	10 grams fat	6.4 grams fat
3 teaspoons fat	2 teaspoons fat	1 teaspoon fat

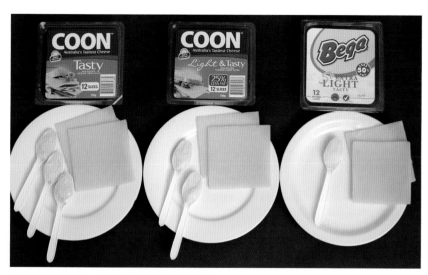

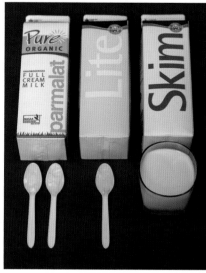

2. Milk 300 ml serve

Full fat	Lite	Skim
3.4 per cent fat	1.4 per cent fat	0
2 teaspoons	1 teaspoon	0

Step 5. Watch those fatty chips

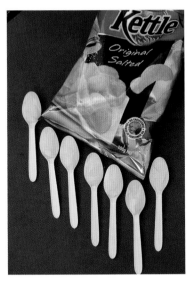

Kettle Original Salted 100 grams
34.6 grams fat (7 teaspoons)

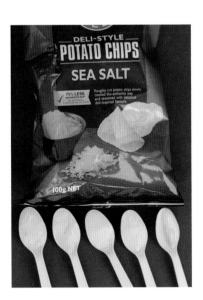

Red Rock Deli Potato Chips Sea Salt 100 grams (75 per cent less saturated fat) 22.5 grams fat (4.5 teaspoons)

Step 6. Watch meat pies and pasties, particularly when served with fried chips

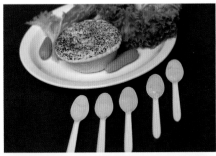

Herbert Adams King Island 210 g meat pie 26 grams fat (5 teaspoons)

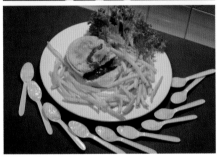

Ordinary common meat pie with McDonald's large serving of fries (130 grams) 51 grams fat (10 teaspoons)

Step 7. Cut back on spreads of butter and margarine if you can—a bad habit indeed. Adding 10 grams of butter or margarine to a slice of bread doubles your caloric intake.

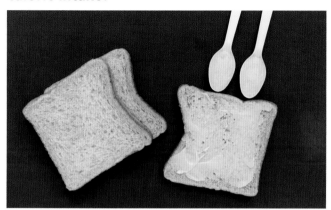

1 Slice of bread plus 2 teaspoons of butter/margarine is equal to 2 'Bread Slice Equivalents'

Most people in the world can't afford to butter their bread. In Western countries it is very common and a very bad habit indeed. Two teaspoons of butter or margarine on four slices of bread a day would result in that person consuming close to 15 kilograms (33 pounds) of unnecessary fat a year. Think of how much that would add up to over a lifetime!

How fattening are nuts?

Nuts are energy-dense foods. They contain some protein (between 2 to 24 per cent), insignificant amounts of carbohydrate (2 to 6 per cent) with the exception of chestnuts (36 per cent) but are very rich in oils. They contain 49 to 73 per cent mostly of the poly and monounsaturated type and for that reason are high in energy and potentially fattening. A 50 gram serve of roasted cashews is equal to 4 'Bread Slice Equivalents'.

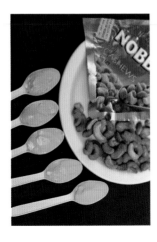

Figure 35: The high content of oil in nuts (cashews 50 gram packet) = 25.6 grams fat/oil = 5 teaspoons

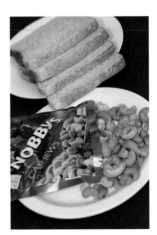

Figure 36: The high caloric content of nuts. 50 grams of cashews is equal to four 'Bread Slice Equivalents'

Because of their insignificant carbohydrate content, when eaten as treats in small amounts, nuts would have a low Glycemic Load (GL)—not having much of an effect on your blood sugars.

> Nuts are high in calories and potentially fattening but do not significantly raise blood sugars partly because they are very low in carbohydrate

How fattening are seeds?

Seeds, like nuts, are energy-dense foods and for a good reason. The seeds of most plants contain oils that serve as a high energy source for new seedlings. Like a hen's egg, a plant seed must contain enough energy for sprouting the first roots, stems and leaves. This occurs until the new plant is sufficiently grown, independent and capable of drawing nutrients from the soil, sun and air for photosynthesis.

Seeds are packed with nutrients and like nuts, are also rich in poly and monounsaturated oils including essential fatty acids. Seeds contain anything up to 50 per cent oil and are potentially fattening. If you do not have a weight problem, they are, like nuts, an excellent way to obtain healthy oils in your diet and are also low in carbohydrate and when eaten in small amounts as snacks would have an insignificant effect on your blood sugars.

Seeds, like nuts, are high in calories and potentially fattening but do not significantly raise blood sugars partly because they are very low in carbohydrate

How fattening are avocados?

Avocados are also energy-dense foods and potentially fattening. They are also rich in poly and monounsaturated oils. They contain anything between 11 to 39 per cent oil according to season, 4.2 per cent protein and hardly any carbohydrate at all. Because they contain minimum carbohydrate they do not affect your blood sugars directly. You can eat avocados but only in moderation if weight is an issue because of their high-energy content.

Avocados, like seeds and nuts, are high in calories and potentially fattening. They do not raise blood sugars because they contain minimal carbohydrate.

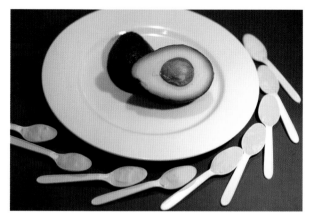

Figure 37: The high content of oil in avocados (9 teaspoons in a 250 gram avocado)

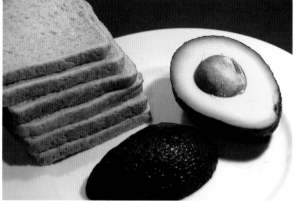

Figure 38: The high caloric content of avocados. One 250 gram avocado is equal to 6 'Bread Slice Equivalents'

So a few slithers of avocado added to your salad to give it taste or using avocado on your bread instead of margarine or butter is unlikely to make you fat. Sitting down to half an avocado for an entrée is another story. Similarly, a few almonds or walnuts, eaten as a healthy mid-morning or afternoon snack instead of biscuits with cheese or dips, or instead of those salty fatty chips are a healthy alternative. Adding a few almonds or sunflower seeds to your cereal in the morning, or a few walnuts or pine nuts to a tossed green salad, is unlikely to make you fat. However, large bowls of salty roasted nuts or pumpkin seeds washed down with several glasses of wine or beer may.

What about extra virgin olive oil?

Extra virgin olive oil, like all oils, is a very energy-dense food because it is made up almost entirely of fatty acids. But it has many other excellent qualities compared to most, if not all oils on the market today. It has not been refined or processed by chemicals and heat. Unlike other oils (safflower, sunflower, corn etc) on your super-market shelf that are extracted from hard seeds, it is easily extracted from the soft flesh of whole, ripe, undamaged fruit.

The freshly harvested olives are put in porous hessian bags and simply cold pressed to extract the green thick oil without the use of solvents or heat—preserving the natural quality of the fatty acids. It is unrefined oil that still contains many natural factors unique to olives known to protect against cardiovascular disease.

> Cold pressed extra virgin olive oil is the only mass marketed oil on your supermarket shelf that has not been processed

This oil has been part of the Mediterranean diet for centuries. It is increasingly becoming the oil of choice worldwide.

I have fond memories of the harvest in my village in Lebanon and of the olive oil mills with their distinct odour wafting in the fresh cold mountainous air. I have lasting memories of my dad and my great uncle at the mills dipping their freshly baked bread in this thick green nectar of the gods. The olive tree in my part of the world is sacred and nothing is wasted. The caked residue after extracting the fine oil is packed in paper bags and used for fuel in winter. The poor quality oil extracted from damaged and shrunken fruits is used to make soap by the village locals.

Cold pressed extra virgin olive oil is the only oil of choice in my household. Unlike extra virgin olive oil, refined olive oil is like most oils on your supermarket shelf. It has suffered significant nutrient losses through industrial processes like degumming, refining, bleaching and deodorising where many of the natural components of the oil are removed. These by the way, are not labeled 'non virgin' in your local supermarket but could be labeled 'pure olive oil' or 'light olive oil'.

I do not get my essential fatty acids from extra virgin olive oil as it is a poor source of these. I get them from fish, seeds (sunflower) and nuts.

> If you have a weight problem, then extra virgin olive oil, nuts, seeds and avocados in the diet should be somewhat restricted

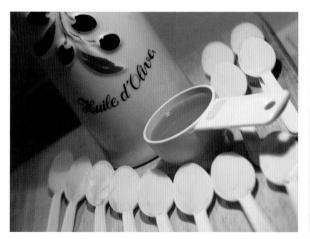

Figure 39: The pure fat content of oil. A quarter of a cup of any oil (60 mls/2 fluid ounces/4 tablespoons) is the equivalent of 12 teaspoons of fat

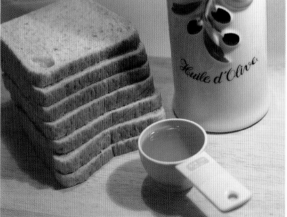

Figure 40: The high caloric density of oil. A quarter of a cup of oil (60 mls/2 fluid ounces/4 tablespoons) is equal to 7 'Bread Slice Equivalents'.

2. The effect of fats and oils on your blood fat levels

As far as we know, there is no difference between one fat/oil and another when it comes to your weight status, however there is a difference when it comes to the effects these fats and oils have on your blood cholesterol levels.

> Not all fats and oils affect your cholesterol

Animal fats and your cholesterol levels

The fats that raise your cholesterol levels most are the hard saturated animal fats not the vegetable oils. Those fats that are solid at room temperature have the most damaging effect. Saturated fats that come from ruminant animals that regurgitate their food like cows and sheep are generally the worst because unlike most other animals we eat that have only one stomach these animals have four, the largest of which is known as a rumen. A rumen is a large fermentation vat full of bugs that convert vegetable oils in the plants they eat to saturated fats. It is really like a margarine factory where plant oils are chemically converted into harder fats. These animals also produce very small amounts of trans fatty acids naturally during this process.

To lower your cholesterol levels you need to reduce or even avoid dairy fats, the fats off your lamb chop or beef steak and any processed product cooked with animal fats such as fast foods. Make sure you stick to low-fat, if not skim milk dairy products if you have a cholesterol problem. Also make sure your meats are very lean. Even better, increase the frequency of fish and chicken and lean pork instead.

Remember, as hunter/gatherers and until humans settled and started raising animals about 10,000 years ago, it was unlikely that any dairy products were eaten at all by adults and only wild animals, not the less lean domesticated animals, were eaten. Maybe we still have not evolved to handle these saturated animal fats.

> Saturated fats from ruminant animals (dairy fats and red meat fats) are the worst for someone with a cholesterol problem

In Western societies where activity levels remain rather low, one recommendation that all nutrition authorities and Diabeties Associations agree on is the importance of reducing fat generally and particularly saturated fats in the diet

What are Trans Fatty Acids (TFAs)?

These are relative newcomers to today's diet that are known to be just as damaging as saturated fats in blocking arteries and increasing the risk of cardiovascular disease. Although they are found in our present diet in far smaller amounts than saturated fats, they are potentially a problem with ever-increasing amounts being used in the food processing industry. TFAs are a type of unsaturated fatty acid that can impact on health by adversely raising the bad LDL cholesterol and reducing the good HDL cholesterol which increases the risk of cardiovascular disease (www.heartfoundation.com.au).

Where do TFAs come from?

Low levels of TFAs occur naturally in the fat of dairy products and meat. They are formed in small amounts within the gut of ruminant animals. However, they are largely formed in the food manufacturing industry today. Over the past decade, manufacturers have been pressurised by consumers and health authorities to move away from hard saturated animal fats as they are known to increase the risk of heart disease. So they had to find a way to make vegetable oils take on the characteristics of animal fats, that is remaining solid at room temperature to improve texture and spreadability.

TFAs are largely formed during the process of superheating of vegetable oils under high pressure, in the chemical process of making semi-solid fats from liquid polyunsaturated fatty acids (partial hydrogenation) for use as edible oil spreads, margarine or as shortening for baking. These would be the main products from which we get trans fatty acids today.

TFAs are largely formed during the process of hydrogenation of vegetable oils to be used in our diet as spreads, margarine and shortening

Because TFAs extend the shelf life of processed foods, they are increasingly being used in the food manufacturing industry. Under pressure, some takeaway food chains have reduced the use of saturated fats but instead have been using partially hydrogenated oil, thus introducing TFAs into our diet instead. You would be advised to read labels and suspect that TFAs would be present in any product with 'partially hydrogenated vegetable oil' in the ingredients. Hunter/gatherers would have been spared the worry.

> TFAs would be found in commercial baked goods like cookies, crackers, donuts, croissants, frozen meals like pizzas and fish fingers, snacks like potato and corn chips, instant soups and prepared noodles

Are TFAs identified on labels?
In Australia and New Zealand, manufacturers only have to identify TFAs on the label if they make a nutritional claim about cholesterol, saturated, polyunsaturated, monounsaturated or omega fatty acids.

The effect of fish oils on your blood fats
The judicious consumption of fish a couple of times a week, as part of a healthy diet, is strongly recommended in patients with diabetes. Long chain omega 3 fatty acids—eicosapentaenoic acid (EPA), docosahexaenoic acid (DHA) that are found predominantly in oily fish such as mackerel, herrings, sardines, salmon and tuna and other seafood are known to reduce triglycerides, have anti-inflammatory and cardiovascular benefits. To reduce triglycerides, fish oil tablets, in doses up to 3 grams per day could also be used, not as the first choice of drug, but as second-line agents in patients with Type 2 diabetes.

The effect of plant sterols on your blood fats
Plant sterols are substances with a similar composition to cholesterol that are found in plant-based foods such as vegetables, legumes, fruits, nuts and seeds in small amounts. These sterols naturally lower the absorption of cholesterol from the gut, leading to a modest fall in blood cholesterol levels. So anyone who eats plenty of

these foods would already be taking in a certain amount of sterols.

Today, some margarine spreads are being enriched with these plant sterols and have been found to lower cholesterol levels by around 10 per cent.[118] These include margarines like Logicol™ and Flora Pro-activ.™ These sterols are now finding their way into other products (for example yoghurts) for the same reason.

If you have cholesterol problems, you can replace your normal margarines with one of these but keep the amount down to 3 to 4 teaspoons per day. Additional intakes provide no extra benefit. Remember, like all margarines they are very high in fat. However, today, a reduced fat form Logical Extra Light™ is

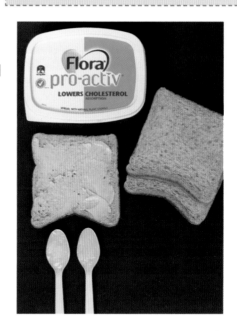

available. It has the same cholesterol—lowering benefits but with half the calories.

The effect of nuts and seeds on your blood fats and heart disease

Research has shown that frequent nut consumers (60 to 150 grams/2 to 5 ounces per week) have a relatively lower risk of heart disease compared with those who rarely ate nuts after accounting for age , smoking and other coronary risk factors.[119] This has also been shown in a Seventh Day Adventist study.[120] There are many reasons for this reduced risk:

1. Nuts are high in polyunsaturated and monounsaturated oils and low in the bad saturated fats.
2. Nuts and seeds contain omega 3 fatty acids like the essential fatty acid, alpha linolenic acid which are lacking in the Western diet. ALA belongs to the same omega 3 family as fish oils. These omega 3 fatty acids are known to reduce the risk of heart disease as previously described.
3. Nuts contain fibre and the anti-oxidant vitamin E that may also help lower cardiovascular risk.

So based on the evidence to date, it is appropriate to include nuts and seeds in a healthy diabetic diet. These are best eaten as nature packaged them- protected from the elements with a natural antioxidant (vitamin E) and a shell or casing that minimises the exposure to the elements of heat, light and air all of which are known to cause fats to spoil or go rancid.

For those who are overweight, professional dietary help from an Accredited Practising Dietitian (APD) on how to plan healthy diets that include nuts is recommended.

> To include seeds and nuts in your diet, their high energy (caloric) content has to be taken into account to help you achieve your target weight

What if you had a cholesterol but not a weight problem?

Then you can get away with having more natural oils found in nuts, seeds, avocados and olives. These are ideal for someone who has already reached their target weight and still losing but trying to stop further weight loss.

Studies have shown that if your weight is fine and have more monounsaturated oil at the expense of carbohydrate in the diet, that overall diabetes control does not deteriorate or may even improve. Blood sugars improve understandably as carbohydrate that ends up as sugar in the blood, is being reduced somewhat in the diet. Blood fats also improve slightly or remain unaffected because these vegetable oils do not have an unfavourable effect on blood fats.[121] Admittedly, these studies have been short term and the long-term effects, particularly on weight status, have not been adequately studied.

If you were active enough, could you get away with eating animal fats?

Well, maybe. There is a tribe in sub-Saharan and West Africa called the Fulani. They are semi-nomadic pastoralists who herd cattle and consume a diet rich in meat and dairy products. Despite their high saturated fat diet, the Fulani adults have normal blood cholesterol profiles indicative of a low risk of heart and blood vessel disease. This is believed to be because their high activity level and low energy intake generally keep them lean.

Another example is the Amish of Pennsylvania in the United States. They have a traditional Northern European diet that is high in fats and protein, so they have not really adopted the lower cholesterol, lower fat diets that much of the more modern Western world has. In spite of that, their cholesterol levels are lower than the general population, their triglyceride levels are very low and they tend to have high HDL levels. Again, it is believed by scientists at the medical School, University of Maryland, Baltimore, that as farmers, it's their physical activity and fitness level that is protecting them from cardiovascular disease.

FATS and OILS—SUMMARY
- Reduce total fat in your diet to help lose any extra weight
- Focus particularly on reducing saturated hard animal fats from full fat dairy and fatty red meat
- Reduce Trans Fatty Acids usually found in manufactured products (margarines, shortenings etc)
- Use cold-pressed extra virgin olive oil for your allowance of 3 to 4 teaspoons/day
- Try to eat fish at least twice per week for those Omega 3 fatty acids

---

FATS AND OILS in the hunter/gatherer's diet
- Much less than what we eat today as foods were eaten in their natural unprocessed, unrefined form (nuts, seeds etc)
- Saturated fat intake would be low as wild animals are lean and are cooked straight on the fire
- The 'essential fats' needed by the body in small amounts would easily be obtained from nuts and seeds and fish
- Seafood, with the good Omega 3 fatty acids, would be a major part of the diet, in communities living next to the sea

12: Red Light Foods = Stop ALCOHOL

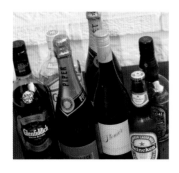

The relationship between alcohol consumption, diabetes and the Metabolic Syndrome remains unclear. Some studies have shown improvements in insulin sensitivity with moderate alcohol consumption in middle-aged women.[122,123] There is also some evidence to suggest a 30 per cent reduction in the incidence of diabetes in those who drink alcohol in moderation.[124] On the other hand, lifetime drinking patterns have also been significantly associated with decreased insulin sensitivity and Metabolic Syndrome risk factors[125] and heavy alcohol consumption has been associated with an increased incidence of diabetes.[126] There is no evidence that hunter/gatherers distilled alcoholic beverages.[34] It would seem that alcohol is yet again a relative newcomer to our diet.

How are alcoholic beverages made?

All alcoholic beverages are made from two basic ingredients: a source of sugar or carbohydrate such as barley, malt, wheat, rice, potato, grapes or plums and yeast. The yeast uses up the sugar source yielding ethanol and gases in a fermentation process. A residual amount of sugar may also be found in the final product depending on the length of the fermentation process; the longer the process the less sugar. For example, wine is made from a variety of grapes. The characteristics of the wine like colour, taste, amount of alcohol and sugar in the final product would depend on the source, the type and colour of the grape and the length of the fermentation process to name a few factors. The longer the fermentation process the less sugar and the drier the product. That's why we have sweet wines and dry wines.

Alcoholic beverages contain ethyl alcohol and a varying amount of residual sugar

1. The effect of alcohol on your weight

Calories in alcoholic drinks come from both the alcohol and residual sugar content. Calories obtained from ethyl alcohol (7 Calories, 29 kilojoules per gram) and carbohydrate (4 Calories, 16.7 kilojoules per gram) are important to the weight watcher. Although the body tends to burn up the alcohol first because it treats it as a toxin, alcohol helps stack away any extra calories from dietary fat, carbohydrate and protein, hence the common beer belly. Alcoholic beverages contain varying amounts of sugar and alcohol. Aside from the calories provided by ethyl alcohol (ethanol) and sugar, these beverages are of no nutritional value. For this reason they are classified as *empty calories*.

Table 16. The alcohol and sugar content of different alcoholic beverages		
Beverage	Alcohol content %	Sugar content %
Beer, conventional	3.5–6.0	2–3
stouts	7.0	2–4
Low alcohol	2–2.7	1.5–2.5
Diet Beers	3.6	0.5–0.8
Cider	5	1–5
Alcoholic soda	4.5	6
Table wine, dry	8–14	1–5
Table wine, sweet	8–14	5–10
Sherry, dry	16–20	1–5
Sherry, sweet	16–20	5–15
Port	17–20	10–20
Spirits (brandy, rum, gin, whisky	35–40	0
liqueurs	35–40	20–30

Alcoholic strengths vary considerably. For example, beer contains between 2 to 6 per cent alcohol, while wines vary from 8 to 14 per cent and spirits between 35 to 40 per cent. The sugar content also varies from less than 1 per cent in 'diet beers' to 1 to 5 per cent for dry wines, 5 to 10 per cent for sweet wines and 20 to 30 per cent for liqueurs.

We now use the concept of a 'standard drink' which is defined as the amount of beverage containing 10 grams of pure ethyl alcohol. You can see that common standard servings of different beverages contain roughly 65 to 110 Calories (272 to 460 kilojoules). So whenever you have two glasses of wine or two nips of whisky or two midis of beer you are taking in two 'Standard Drinks' and somewhere between 130-200 Calories (544 to 837 kilojoules) or 2 to 3 'Bread Slice Equivalents' depending on the sugar content of the drink.

> A 'standard drink' is defined as the amount of beverage containing 10 grams of ethyl alcohol

Consuming excess alcohol may result in weight gain and potential problems with obesity[127, 128] whereas those who drink moderately are at no greater risk.[129]

Table 17. A 'standard drink' of different alcoholic beverages (containing 10 grams of alcohol)

Beverage	Volume mls (ounces)	Kilojoules/Calories
Beer 1 midi (2/3 can)	280 (9.5)	364/87
Beer (1 can) reduced alcohol	375 (12.5)	460/110
Low alcohol beer (1 can)	375 (12.5)	315/75
Wine, dry, (1 glass)	120 (4)	335/80
Champagne (1 flute)	120 (4)	325/78
Port or Sherry (1 glass)	60 (2)	380/90
Spirits (1 nip)	30 (1)	272/65

There is evidence that moderate alcohol intake can increase triglycerides and HDL cholesterol in the non-diabetic population. However, there is no direct evidence to date that alcohol alters the blood fat profile in people with Type 2 diabetes[50] but some studies show that moderate alcohol consumption reduces the incidence of heart disease.[130]

3. The effect of alcohol on your blood sugar levels (hypoglycemia)

Alcohol can cause a drop in blood sugars and cause hypos. However, this is only likely to happen in those on insulin. This can be avoided by not drinking on an empty stomach but with food. It is also recommended that people with diabetes on insulin who plan to drive abstain from drinking because of possible impaired cognitive function.[131]

> Alcohol can cause a 'hypo' or low blood sugar in those on insulin and for that reason should be taken with food

What are recommended intakes of alcohol for people with diabetes?
Alcohol is an important and pleasurable part of our diet and there is no reason why, in moderation, it cant be part of a healthy balanced diabetic diet.

A maximum of two 'standard drinks' per day for males and one for females are acceptable recommendations as part of a balanced diet.

> A maximum of one 'standard drink' per day for females and two 'standard drinks' for males are acceptable recommendations for people with diabetes

ALCOHOL—SUMMARY
- Alcohol in moderation may be enjoyed by people with diabtes
- People should be aware of the caloric value of alcoholic drinks: one standard drink has a minimum energy value of 70 Calories (293 kilojoules) or one 'Bread Slice Equivalent'
- Those on insulin and some diabetic tablets should be aware of the blood sugar lowering (hypoglycemic) effect of alcohol and for that reason should not drink on an empty stomach
- One standard drink (a glass of wine, a midi of beer, or a nip of spirit) for females and two standards for males per day is an acceptable recommendation

ALCOHOL in the hunter/gatherer's diet
- There is no evidence that hunter/gatherer's distilled alcohol
- Alcohol is a newcomer to the human diet

13: Your diabetes plan

Think of yourself as a hunter/gatherer in your journey to good health

It is not possible to totally replicate the hunter/gatherer's way of life today. But, it would be wise of you to use this model as a template for changing your lifestyle to help treat and even prevent diabetes and its cardiovascular complications. Yes, the time has come to make the necessary lifestyle changes to help realign your way of life with that of your ancient ancestors. I want you to think of yourself as a hunter/gatherer when you are:

» **Shopping:** Remember, stick to the unprocessed unrefined foods. Forget about the cans and packages generally and try and go for the fresh foods. Plenty of green leafy vegetables, low-GI fruits, starchy vegetables and multi-grain breads, fresh lean fish, chicken, pork, veal, seafood and meats.
» **Cooking:** Try not to add much oil or fat, particularly animal fat. Use cold pressed extra virgin olive oil.
» **Eating:** Small and often to help control your blood sugars. Remember this ideal plate of half greens, quarter protein and quarter low-GI carbohydrates.
» **Sitting pressing buttons:** Try to get those legs moving for at least 30 minutes a day to help your overall diabetes control.

If your ancient ancestors did not do it then think twice

Elements of your 'Ideal Diabetic Diet'

How many calories should you be on?

» If you are of normal weight with no extras around the waistline, then your recommended energy or caloric intake from food should remain the same. For example, if you normally consume 1700 Calories (7113 kilojoules), you will most likely be prescribed the same by your Accredited Practising Dietitian (APD).

> If you are of normal weight you will be prescribed the caloric intake you normally eat

» If you are overweight or obese, particularly around the waistline, then limiting your caloric intake is probably the single most important dietary change you need to make along with increased activity. You will most likely have to compromise with the amount of carbohydrate and move to low-GI forms in order to reduce the Glycemic Load (GL) at each meal. Protein intakes may need to be reduced also. You could increase your greens at the expense of carbohydrates and proteins to speed up that process. Remember, the greens are very low in calories. See Appendix C for the caloric content of some commonly eaten foods expressed in 'Bread Slice Equivalents'. A moderate decrease in caloric balance (500 to 1000 Calories/day; 2092 to 4184 kilojoules) will result in a slow but steady weight loss of half to one kilogram (1 to 2 pounds) of body fat per week, which is a healthy rate of weight loss. For most patients, weight loss diets should supply around 1000 to 1200 Calories (4184 to 5021 kilojoules) per day for females and 1400 to 1600 Calories (5858 to 6694 kilojoules) for males (see Meal Plans No 1 and 2 below).

> If you are overweight then limiting your caloric intake is the single most important dietary recommendation

What about the quality of food you should be eating?

The quality of your food will most likely have to change to control your diabetes and Metabolic Syndrome risk factors like weight, blood sugars, blood fats and blood pressure. Authorities recommend that people generally, including those with diabetes, consume a diet where carbohydrate (preferably low-GI) contributes 40 to 55 per cent of total energy, protein 15 to 30 per cent and fats (mostly mono and polyunsaturated) 25 to 30 per cent. Although studies have tried to find the optimal combination of protein, fat and carbohydrate, it is unlikely that any one combination meets everyone's needs, let alone likes and dislikes. The best combination is the one that best suits your individual circumstances. A little less carbohydrate and more protein if you are a meat eater or vice versa if you are a carbohydrate eater is all acceptable. Remember, you have to live with this for the rest of your life—with additional treats of course.

> Your diet should be tailored to your individual requirements likes and dislikes by an Accredited Practising Dietitian (APD)

Consulting your Accredited Practising Dietitian (APD)

Dietitians, working in the area of diabetes management, are clinically trained for Medical Nutrition Therapy (MNT) and can work out your individual lifestyle and dietary needs. I strongly advise all patients to consult an Accredited Practising Dietitian (APD). Many, but not all, patients diagnosed with pre-diabetes/diabetes are now seeking advice mainly for the following reasons:

» Dietitians are increasingly being recognised as the sole authority qualified for Medical Nutrition Therapy.
» Doctors are increasingly referring to dietitians.
» There are more available dietitians in private practice.
» All private health funds cover private consults.
» The public health system in Australia (Medicare) does not cover private nutrition consults. However, recently there has been a glimmer of hope for patients with a chronic disease like diabetes who are not privately insured. The Australian Health Insurance Commission has introduced incentives for

General Practitioners to refer to APDs as part of a Health Care Plan that has proven to be successful and a welcome change. Discuss that with your GP for you might be entitled to five sessions per year.

> If you are not privately insured, ask your doctor to set up a Care Plan for you so you can be referred to a dietitian under the public health system

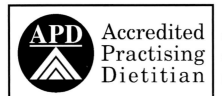

APDs in Australia are listed in the Yellow Pages and on the Dietitians' Association of Australia website (www.daa.asn.au). A doctor's referral is preferable but not required for reimbursements from private health funds. Members of the Dietitians' Association are bound by a professional code of conduct and APDs are required to participate in a mandatory continuing professional development program.

Following an individual assessment, the dietitian will prescribe a diet tailored to your individual medical requirements. They may prescribe a set of Carbohydrate Exchanges for each meal and may be for snacks between meals to evenly space the carbohydrate over the day to help control your blood sugars. A Carbohydrate Exchange is described as the amount of carbohydrate food containing 15 grams of carbohydrate.

A typical distribution of Carbohydrate Exchanges for females trying to lose weight is two for each main meal and if any, one for snacks between meals (see Meal Plan No 1). A typical distribution for males trying to lose weight is three for each main meal and, if any, one for snacks between meals (see Meal Plan No 2).

> Carbohydrates at meals/snacks could be reduced even further for some more lean protein in the diet

Table 18. A short list of Exchanges of low-GI carbohydrate foods *

Fruits	Amount
Apples	1 small (125 g/4 oz)
Pears	1 small (150 g/5 oz)
Oranges	1 small (160 g/5 oz)
Peach	1 large (200 g/7 oz)
Grapes	20 medium (100 g/3 oz)
Mango	1 medium (180 g/6 oz)

Starchy vegetables	
Sweet potato	½ cup cooked
Sweet corn	½ cup cooked
Lentils	½ cup cooked
Kidney beans	½ cup cooked

Breads	
Multigrain	1 slice (30 g/1 oz)
Rye	1 slice (30 g)
Black	1 slice (30 g)
Sourdough	1 slice (30 g)

Cereals and biscuits	
Traditional Oats (dry)	¼ cup
Kellogg's All-Bran™	¼ cup
Pasta	½ cup cooked
Basmati rice	$1/3$ cup cooked
Oatmeal biscuits	2

* Each Exchange contains 15 grams of carbohydrate

Meal Plan No 1: A typical meal plan for **women** with Type 2 diabetes trying to lose weight (1200 Calories/5020 kilojoules with 50 per cent carbohydrate)

Breakfast

Dry oats	¼ cup dry
Pear	1 small
Low-fat milk	From allowance*
Tea/coffee	

Morning tea

Apple /orange	1 small
Tea/coffee	

Lunch (light)

Multigrain bread	2 slices (30g/1 oz each)
Salmon/tuna/chicken/ham	30 grams (1 oz)
Salad (tomato, lettuce etc)	As much as possible
Margarine	From allowance*
Tea/coffee	

Afternoon tea

Peach/nectarine etc	1 large
Tea/coffee	

Dinner (cooked)

Fish/chicken/veal/beef/lamb (lean)	90 g (3 oz)
Sweet potato/basmati rice/pasta	$^2/_3$–1 cup
Free vegetable (salad/stir fry/soup)	Eat freely (at least ½ your plate)

Supper

Oatmeal biscuit	2
Tea/coffee	

*Daily allowance: Low-fat milk 400 ml (13 fl oz), margarine or olive oil 3 teaspoons.

Carbohydrate: 2 exchanges per meal; 1 exchange for each snack

Protein: 120 g/4 oz per day

Free Vegetables: Eat freely

Meal Plan No 2: A typical meal plan for **men** with Type 2 diabetes trying to lose weight (1500 Calories/6276 kilojoules with 50 per cent carbohydrate)

Breakfast

Dry oats	½ cup dry
Pear	1 small
Low-fat milk	From allowance*
Tea/coffee	

Morning tea

Apple /orange	1 small
Tea/coffee	

Lunch (light)

Multigrain bread	2 slices (30 g/1 oz each)
Salmon/tuna/chicken/	60 grams (2 oz)
Salad (tomato, lettuce etc)	As much as possible
Orange	1 small
Margarine	From allowance*
Tea/coffee	

Afternoon tea

Peach/nectarine etc	1 large
Tea/coffee	

Dinner (cooked)

Fish/chicken/veal/beef/lamb (lean)	120 g/4 oz
Sweet potato/basmati rice/pasta	⅔–1 cup
Fruit	Small apple
Free vegetable	
(Salad/stir fry/soup/steamed)	Eat freely (at least ½ your plate)
Tea/coffee	

Supper

Oatmeal biscuit	2
Tea/coffee	

*Daily allowance: Low-fat milk 400 ml (13 fl oz), margarine or olive oil 4 teaspoons.
Carbohydrate: 3 exchanges per meal; 1 exchange for each snack
Protein: 180 g/6 oz per day
Free Vegetables: Eat freely

Breakfasts: reduced glycemic load

Breakfast is an important meal of the day for all. My general experience is that those who miss breakfast and eat most of their food in the evening are the ones more likely to be struggling with their weight. As the old saying goes 'breakfast like a king, lunch like a prince and dine like a pauper'.

Most people with diabetes are on some medication to help lower blood sugars and that is another reason not to miss breakfast. You should not take your tablets or insulin on an empty stomach for risk of low blood sugars or hypoglycemia.

Breakfast should consist of some low-GI cereal or bread or fruit with a cup of tea or coffee made with low/reduced fat milk.

Meal Plan 1 for *Women* trying to lose weight
Some breakfast options containing 2 Carbohydrate Exchanges (30 g/1 oz of carbohydrate) each:

- » 1 exchange of traditional oats (¼ cup dry) plus 1 small pear. Milk from your daily allowance (400 ml/13 fl oz).
- » 1 exchange of traditional oats (¼ cup dry) plus 1 slice (30 g/1 oz) of low-GI bread (Burgen™ Soy and Linseed) some margarine from your allowance with vegemite
- » 2 exchanges of traditional oats (½ cup dry) eaten as is or cooked plus low-fat milk or diet flavoured yoghurt
- » 2 slices (60 g/2 oz) of low-GI bread (multigrain, soy and linseed, sourdough etc) with some margarine out of your allowance plus some Vegemite, tomato or asparagus or low-calorie/joule jam
- » 2 low-GI fruits cut up as in a fruit salad plus some low-fat flavoured yoghurt
- » Kellogg's All Bran™ ¼ cup plus a small pear plus low-fat milk

Tea/coffee artificially sweetened or with 1 teaspoon of sugar. You may have some protein such as low-fat cheese or an egg out of your daily allowance of protein (120g/4oz) for breakfast.

Meal Plan 2 for *Men* trying to lose weight

Some breakfast options containing 3 Carbohydrate Exchanges (45g/1½ oz) each:

» 1 exchange from traditional oats (¼ cup dry) plus 1 slice (30g/1oz) of low-GI bread (Burgen™ Soy and Linseed) plus a small orange

» 2 exchanges of traditional oats (½ cup dry) eaten as is or cooked plus low-fat milk plus a small pear

» 2 slices (60g/2oz) of low-GI bread (soy and linseed, sourdough etc) with some margarine out of your allowance plus some Vegemite, tomato or asparagus or low-calorie/joule jam plus a small size apple

» 2 low-GI fruits cut up as in a fruit salad plus some low-fat flavoured yoghurt and 1 slice (30g/1oz) of low-GI sourdough bread with Vegemite and margarine from your allowance

» Kellogg's All Bran™ (¼ cup dry) plus a small pear plus low-fat milk plus 1 slice (30g/1oz) of low-GI Burgen™ Rye bread with peanut butter or Vegemite

Tea/coffee are free with milk from your allowance. Use an artificial sweetener or 1 teaspoon of sugar. You may have some protein such as low-fat cheese or an egg out of your daily allowance of protein (180g/6oz) for breakfast.

Snacks: Reduced glycemic load

These include morning tea, afternoon tea and supper. If you are on diet alone for your diabetes you need not take snacks between meals as you are at no risk of having low blood sugars or hypos. If you are on medication to lower your blood sugars, you may or may not need to have snacks between meals. (see Chapter 8, page 133). If you are struggling to lose weight with snacks between meals, you may want to drop some of these snacks and reduce your blood sugar tablets to prevent having low blood sugars or hypos.

Meal Plans 1 and 2 for both *Women* and *Men* trying to lose weight
Some snack options containing 1 Carbohydrate Exchange (15 grams of carbohydrate) each:
  » 1 exchange of low-GI fruit (apple, pear, orange, peach, plum, nectarine, mango). You may add some low-fat yoghurt as in a fruit salad
  » I slice (30g/1oz) of low-GI bread (multigrain, sourdough) with margarine from your allowance. Vegemite, low-calorie/joule jam.
  » 2 oatmeal biscuits

Tea and coffee are free with milk from your allowance. Use an artificial sweetner or a small teaspoon of sugar.

Lunches: Reduced glycemic load

One of the most common causes of excess caloric intake and weight problems in my experience is patients partaking in two main meals per day. Many working men and women tend to have a fast takeaway meal (Thai, Chinese etc) at lunch and then have another main meal at night with their family. I strongly advise patients against that if weight is an issue. You either have a light meal at lunch such as sandwiches and a main meal at night or vice a versa. This can significantly reduce your caloric intake and help you lose weight.

Meal Plan 1 for *Women* trying to lose weight

Some lunch options containing 2 Carbohydrate Exchanges (30g/1oz of carbohydrate) each:

» 2 slices (60g/2oz) of low-GI bread (soy and linseed, sourdough etc) in a sandwich with some margarine out of your allowance plus 30g (1oz) of protein (smoked salmon, canned tuna, ham, corned beef, turkey, chicken, egg) with plenty of free vegetables.

» 2 low-GI fruits cut up as in a fruit salad plus some low-fat flavoured yoghurt out of your allowance of 400 mls (13fl oz) of low-fat milk/yoghurt

» A free vegetable soup with 2 slices (60g/2oz) of low-GI bread

Tea and coffee are free with milk from your allowance. Use an artificial sweetener or a small teaspoon of sugar. Drink plenty of water and occasionally, you could have a diet soft drink as they are free of calories and do not affect your blood sugars. It might even keep you awake for the rest of the afternoon!

Meal Plan 2 for *Men* trying to lose weight

Some lunch options containing 3 Carbohydrate Exchanges (45g/1½ oz of carbohydrate) each include:

» 2 slices of low-GI bread (Multigrain, soy and linseed, sourdough etc) with some margarine out of your allowance plus (60 g/2 oz) of protein (tuna, smoked salmon, turkey, ham, reduced-fat cheese) and plenty of free vegetables. 1 exchange of low-GI fruit (strawberries, large peach, small orange, small apple).

» 3 low-GI fruits cut up as in a fruit salad plus some low-fat flavoured yoghurt from your allowance of 400 ml (13 fl oz) of low-fat milk/yoghurt per day

Tea and coffee are free with milk from your allowance. Use an artificial sweetener or a small teaspoon of sugar. Drink plenty of water and occasionally, you could have a diet soft drink as they are free of calories and do not affect your blood sugars. It might even keep you awake for the rest of the afternoon!

Dinners: Reduced glycemic load

For people who are working, dinner is often the main meal of the day. For retirees who have plenty of time on their hands, lunch can often be the main meal. I recommend that you design your main meal for the day, whether it be lunch or dinner, around the Plate Model with plenty of free vegetables (½ plate) moderate amounts of low-GI carbohydrate (¼ plate) and lean protein (¼ plate).

Meal Plan 1 for *Women* trying to lose weight
Some dinner options containing 2 Carbohydrate Exchanges (30g/1oz of carbohydrate) each:
Carbohydrate: ²/₃ cup of boiled basmati rice or 1 cup of cooked pasta or sweet potato
Protein: 90g/3oz of lean fish, seafood, chicken, pork, veal, beef or lamb.
Free vegetables: Half plate of stir fried vegetables, soup, salads or steamed vegetables.

Tea and coffee are free with milk from your allowance. Use an artificial sweetener or a small teaspoon of sugar. Drink plenty of water and occasionally, you could have a diet soft drink as they are free of calories and do not affect your blood sugars. You might want to have a glass of wine occasionally with your dinner.

Meal Plan 2 for *Men* trying to lose weight
Some dinner options containing 3 Carbohydrate Exchanges (45g/1½ oz of carbohydrate) each:
Carbohydrate: 1 cup of boiled basmati rice or 1½ cups cooked pasta or sweet potato
Protein: 120 g/4 oz of lean fish, seafood, chicken, pork, veal, beef or lamb
Free vegetables: Half plate of stir fried vegetables, soup, salads or steamed vegetables.

Tea and coffee are free with milk from your allowance. Use an artificial sweetener or a small teaspoon of sugar. Drink plenty of water and occasionally, you could have a diet soft drink as they are free of calories and do not affect your blood sugars. You might want to have 1–2 glasses of wine occasionally with your dinner.

APPENDIX A

How to calculate your Body Mass Index (BMI)

BMI is used to determine your weight status. It is simply calculated by dividing your weight in kilograms (Kgs) by the square of your height in metres (m²). For example I weigh 70 kilograms and my height is 1.72 metres. My BMI is calculated as follows:

$$BMI = 70/(1.72)^2 = 70/2.96 = 23.6$$

According to the table below I am within the normal weight range

BMI	Weight Status
<20	Underweight
20–25	Normal
25–30	Overweight
30–35	Grade 1 Obesity
35–40	Grade 2 Obesity
>40	Grade 3 Obesity

APPENDIX B

How to measure your waistline correctly

It is easy to incorrectly measure your waistline with a tape. For an accurate measurement:

» **First:** measure with the minimum of clothes—or better still no clothing at all
» **Second:** measure at the halfway point between the top of your hipbone and your lowest rib. This will be roughly in line with your belly button.
» **Third:** The tape measure should be snug and not tight.

APPENDIX C

The caloric content of commonly eaten foods expressed in 'Bread Slice Equivalents'

As a weight watcher it is important to realise that the single most important dietary factor is the energy in your food expressed in Calories or kilojoules. Yes- carbohydrates are important as you have diabetes, fats and types of fats are important as they are high in energy and could affect you blood fats, but total calories is most important. Because most people cannot relate to calories, I have tried to simplify the concept by expressing the energy content of foods in what I call 'Bread Slice Equivalents' defined as the calories found in a standard 30 gram slice of bread (70 Calories/293 kilojoules). I hope this will be an eye opener for you as much as it has been for many of my patients. For comparison, I have included foods from the different tiers of the Healthy Food Pyramid starting with the least fattening Green Light Foods (example lettuce) all the way up to the Red Light Foods (soft drinks to the most concentrated source of calories in food which is pure oil).

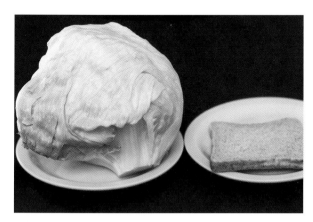

One medium lettuce is equal to
1 'Bread Slice Equivalent'

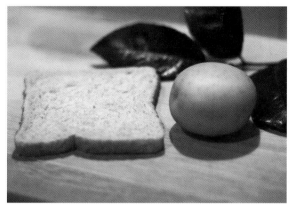

A small 75 gram potato is equal to
1 'Bread Slice Equivalent'

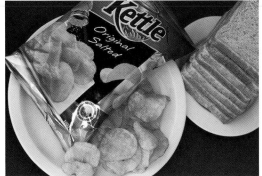

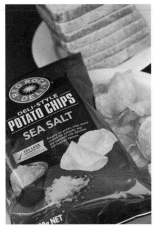

A 100 gram packet of 75 per cent less saturated fat chips is equal to 7 'Bread Slice Equivalents'

A 100 gram packet of Kettle chips is equal to 8 'Bread Slice Equivalents'

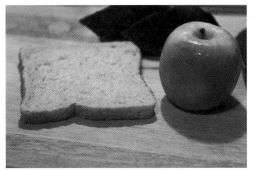

A small 125 gram apple is equal to 1 'Bread Slice Equivalent'

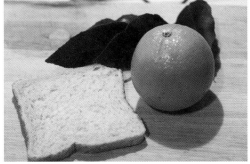

A small size orange (160 grams) is equal to 1 'Bread Slice Equivalent'

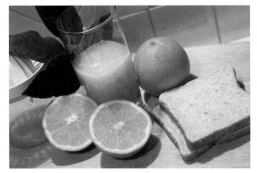

The freshly squeezed juice of two small size oranges (160 grams each) is equal to 2 'Bread Slice Equivalents'

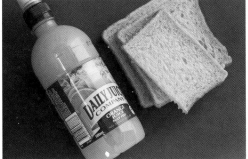

A 500 ml bottle of daily juice (partly fresh and partly reconstituted) is equal to 2.75 'Bread Slice Equivalents'

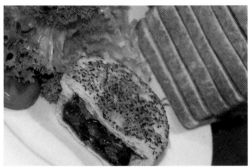

A 210 gram Herbert Adams King Island Meat Pie is equal to 7 'Bread Slice Equivalents'

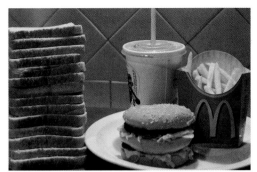

A McValue Meal (A Big Mac, a medium fries, a medium Coke) is equal to 14 'Bread Slice Equivalents'

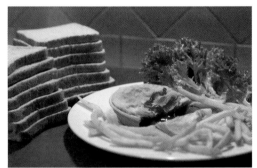

An ordinary Meat Pie and a large (130 gram) serving of finely cut French Fries is equal to 14 'Bread Slice Equivalents'

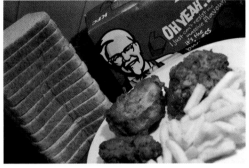

A 'Chicken 'N Chips Pack' containing 3 pieces of chicken and a regular chips is equal to 13 'Bread Slice Equivalents'

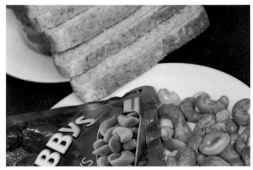

A 50 gram packet of cashews is equal to 4 'Bread Slice Equivalents'

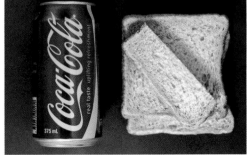

A can of coke (375 mls) is equal to 2.3 'Bread Slice Equivalents'

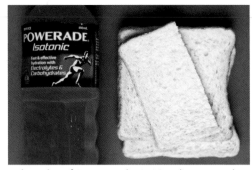

A bottle of Powerade (600 ml) is equal to 2.6 'Bread Slice Equivalents'

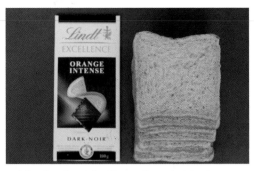

A block of Lindt Chocolate (100 g) is equal to 7 'Bread Slice Equivalents'

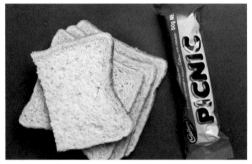

A Picnic bar (50 g) is equal to 3.8 'Bread Slice Equivalents'

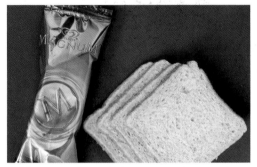

A Magnum Classic ice cream is equal to 4 'Bread Slice Equivalents'

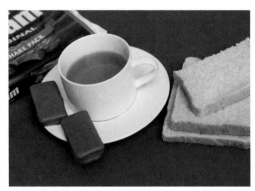

Two Tim Tam™ biscuits are equal to 2¾ 'Bread Slice Equivalents'

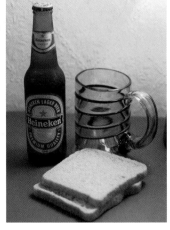

A 330 ml/11fl oz bottle of Heineken Beer of 5 per cent alcohol is equal to 2 'Bread Slice Equivalents'

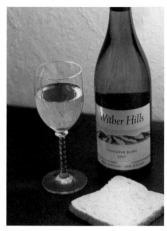

A glass of wine (120 ml/4 fl oz) is equal to 1 'Bread Slice Equivalent'

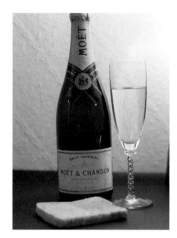

A champagne flute (120 ml/4 fl oz) is equal to 1 'Bread Slice Equivalent'

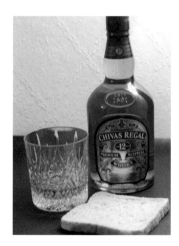

A nip of whiskey (1 fl oz or 30 ml) or any other spirit like gin, rum, vodka is equal to 1 'Bread Slice Equivalent'

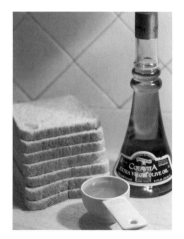

Sixty mls (2 fl oz/ 4 tablespoons/¼ cup) of any oil are equal to 7 'Bread Slice Equivalents'

GLOSSARY

Acanthosis nigricans: Dark patches of skin, usually on the back of the neck associated with severe insulin resistance. Other possible sites for these dark patches include elbows, knees, knuckles, and armpits.

Acarbose: A drug that is used in people with diabetes to lower blood sugars. It works in the small intestine, slowing down the digestion of starch thus reducing blood sugar levels after meals. It is otherwise known as Glucobay™ in Australia and Europe and Precose™ in the United States.

Accredited Practising Dietitian (APD): Is a clinically trained health professional with tertiary (university) qualifications and specialises in Medical Nutrition Therapy (MNT) of dietary—related diseases. They are members of the Dietitians Association of Australia and are bound by a professional code of conduct. APDs are required to participate in a mandatory continuing professional development program.

Acetoacetate: One of three ketones produced by fast breakdown of body fats. It is used as an alternative to glucose as a source of fuel when people with Type 1 diabetes are badly controlled—for example when they don't take their life—saving insulin or when they are sick.

Acetone: One of three ketones produced by fast breakdown of body fats. It is used as an alternative to glucose as a source of fuel when people with Type 1 diabetes are badly controlled—for example when they don't take their life—saving insulin or when they are sick.

Aerobic activity: Activity that consists of 'rhythmic, repeated and continuous movement of the same large muscle groups for at least 10 minute at a time'. Examples include walking, swimming, cycling, running and rowing.

Agricultural Revolution: The period in human history when agriculture and the domestication of animals first emerged as a new way of life replacing hunting and gathering. It started 10,000 years ago in the near East—the Nile valley and Western Asia.

Alpha Linolenic Acid (ALA, 18:3 w3): An 18 carbon fatty acid of the omega 3 series with 3 double bonds. It is the second of the essential fatty acids (EFA) that our body cannot make, requires for good health and must obtain from food. Rich sources include flax and hemp seeds.

Amino acids: The building blocks from which all 'proteins' are made. There are 20 amino acids in nature, 10 of which the body can not make. These 10 are called 'essential amino acids' and need to be obtained from dietary protein foods like meat, chicken, egg, pork, fish and legumes.

Amylopectin: A type of starch where the glucose molecules are arranged in a branched form and for that reason is easy to digest and has a relatively higher GI. That is why jasmine rice has a high GI.

Amylose: A type of starch where the glucose molecules are arranged in a straight line and for that reason is hard to digest and has a low GI. That is why basmati rice has a low GI.

Artificial sweetener: A sweetener used as an alternative to sugar. Examples include Equal™ and Splenda™.

Atherosclerosis: The build up of fatty material in the walls of arteries that can eventually lead to their hardening and blockage. In the heart, this can cause a heart attack, in the brain it can cause a stroke and in the legs it can cause peripheral vascular disease.

Betahydroxybutyrate: One of three ketones produced by the fast breakdown of body fats. It is used as an alternative to glucose as a source of fuel when people with Type 1 diabetes are badly controlled–for example when they don't take their life-saving insulin or when they are sick.

Biguanides: A very successful and common group of drugs used to lower blood sugars in people with diabetes. They help insulin work better. They include drugs like: Metformin™, Diaformin™, Diabex™ and Glucophage™.

Bleaching: The fifth stage in the process of extracting and refining oil from seeds and nuts. It is a filtering process where chlorophyll and the vitamin B-carotene are lost.

Blood fats/lipids: Refer to the concentration of cholesterol (total, HDL, LDL and VLDL) and triglycerides in the blood.

Blood pressure: Refers to vascular pressure i.e. the force exerted by circulating blood on the walls of arteries. Systolic blood pressure is defined as the highest pressure in the arteries, which occurs when the ventricles of the heart contract and the diastolic blood pressure is the lowest pressure at the resting phase of the cardiac cycle. Recommended targets for people with diabetes are 130/85—130 referring to systolic and 80 to diastolic blood pressure.

Bread Slice Equivalent: is the calories found in 1 slice (30g/1oz) of bread and equal to 70 Calories/293 kilojoules which I have used to express the energy value of foods.

Calorie, capital C= kilocalorie (symbol: kcal)): Is a unit of energy defined as the amount of food energy (heat) that will raise one kilogram of water by one degree Celsius. A calorie (small c, symbol: cal) is the amount of energy that will raise one gram of water by one degree Celsius. One Calorie = 1000 calories = one kilocalorie = 4.184 kilojoules (symbol: kJ) (see Joule)

Carbohydrate exchange: The amount of food containing 15 grams of carbohydrate that can be exchanged one for another. Examples: 1 slice of bread, a small apple (125g/4oz), $^1/_3$ cup of cooked rice, ½ cup of cooked pasta.

Cardiovascular disease: A disease caused by narrowing of arteries that feed the heart muscle. This can cause early symptoms such as angina and eventually a heart attack.

Carnivore: An animal that can live on flesh alone. Examples include the lion and the cat.

Central obesity: Excess body fat in the central abdominal area and measured in clinical practice by waistline circumference using a tape measure. It is ethnic specific meaning there are different healthy cut-off points for different ethnic groups. It is strongly associated with fat deep in the abdominal area (visceral fat) that is measured by CT scans and MRIs.

Cerebrovascular disease: A disease caused by blockage of arteries that feed the brain that can eventually cause a stroke.

Degumming: The third stage in the extraction of oil from seeds and nuts. This process removes gums and lecithin, chlorophyll, and minerals like calcium, magnesium and iron from the unrefined oil.

Deodorizing: The sixth stage in the extraction of oil from seeds and nuts. It removes aromatic oils, and molecules that impart bad odours and unpleasant tastes that have been caused by the previous 5 stages of refining. It takes place at a high temperature of 240 – 270 degrees centigrade causing the formation of the bad trans fatty acids. This process also causes the loss of vitamin E—naturally occurring in the oil where it protects the unsaturated fatty acids from oxidation.

Diabesity: A term often used today to describe the strong association of Type 2 diabetes with obesity.

Diabetes (Type 1): The less common form of the disease affecting 10 to 15 per cent of all cases. It is caused when beta cells that produce insulin in the pancreas are attacked by the body's own immune system. It is found generally in young people where daily insulin injections are required for survival.

Diabetes (Type 2): The most common form of diabetes affecting 85 to 90 per cent of all cases. It is a lifestyle disease that can be delayed and may even be prevented with a healthy diet and regular exercise in the early pre-diabetes stage.

Diastolic blood pressure: See Blood pressure.

Dietitian: See Accredited Practising Dietitian (APD).

Disaccharide: A carbohydrate made up of 2 simple sugars linked together. Examples include: lactose the sugar found in milk, maltose otherwise known as malt, and sucrose commonly known as table or cane sugar.

Docosahexaenoic acid (DHA, 22:6 w3): A 22 carbon fatty acid of the omega 3 series with 6 double bonds. It is found in cold water fish and marine animals and can be manufactured in the body from the essential alpha—linolenic acid (18:3 w3). It is commonly taken today in fish oil tablets.

Eicosapentaenoic acid (EPA, 20:5 w3): A 20 carbon polyunsaturated fatty acid of the omega 3 series with 5 double bonds. It is synthesised in the body from the essential fatty acid alpha linolenic acid (ALA, 18:3 w3). EPA is found largely in cold water fish and marine animals. It is commonly taken today in the form of 'fish oil tablets'.

Energy intake: Is the amount of energy obtained from digested food. The total energy is expressed in number of Calories (kilocalories) or kilojoules and calculated from the total fat, protein, carbohydrate and alcohol in your diet.

Energy output: The amount of energy that your body spends. It is the sum of your Basal Metabolic Rate (what you burn resting) plus what you burn up during exercise.

Essential amino acids: Any one of 8 amino acids that the body can not manufacture and must obtain from food. For children, 10 amino acids are essential.

Essential fatty acids (EFA): One of two fatty acids that the body requires, cannot make from other substances and must be acquired from food. These are Linoleic acid (LA: 18:2 w6) and alpha-linolenic acid (ALA 18:3 w3).

Exercise physiologist: A qualified professional within the field of exercise science who has specialised in either health and fitness or exercise rehabilitation.

Fasting blood sugars: Blood sugar levels when tested first thing in the morning after a 10 hour fast overnight.

Fibrates: A class of drugs known to correct abnormal blood fats commonly found in diabetes and the Metabolic Syndrome. It mainly lowers triglycerides and raises the good HDL cholesterol. It includes drugs like Gemfibrozil (Lopid ™) and Fenofibrate (Lipidil™).

Fructose: A simple sugar (monosaccharide) otherwise known as fruit sugar. It is estimated to be twice as sweet as sucrose (table sugar). It is found in combination with glucose and sucrose (table sugar) in fruits. It has a very low GI relative to glucose.

Functional foods: foods fresh or processed thought to have medicinal properties with health benefits beyond their nutrient content. Example: Probiotics and the beneficial effect they have on gut flora.

Genetically Modified (GM) foods: Also known as genetically engineered foods. These are foods that have had their genes modified or slightly altered to impart a certain benefit to the plant: to resist certain bugs, to handle cold climate, to increase production, to increase shelf life etc.

Gestational diabetes: A temporary form of the disease that occurs during pregnancy due to hormonal changes that prevents insulin that is normally produced by the body from doing its job. Normal insulin and blood sugar levels are generally restored post delivery. Women with gestational diabetes have an increased risk of developing Type 2 diabetes in the future.

Glitazones: A group of drugs used to lower blood sugars by helping insulin work better. They include drugs like Avandia™ (Rosiglitazone) and Actos™ (Pioglitazone) which are known to cause fluid retention and weight gain in some people.

Glucometer: A machine available for patients to test blood sugars at home.

Glucagon: A hormone produced by specialised cells in the pancreas to mobilize stores of glycogen (sugar) in the liver and muscle to prevent blood sugars from suddenly dropping too low and causing hypoglycemia.

Gluconeogenesis: The process of synthesising glucose from muscle protein when glycogen stores become depleted upon starvation or prolonged endurance exercise like marathon running.

Glycated Haemoglobin (HbA1c): Also known as A1C is a routine test that reflects blood sugar levels over the previous 2 to 3 months. Normal levels are between 4 and 6 per cent but in clinical practice a target of less than 7 per cent is considered adequate.

Glycemic Index (GI): A rating of carbohydrate foods based on their effect on blood sugars. You have 'low = less than 55', 'medium = 56–69' and 'high = > 70' GI foods—the low-GI foods raising blood sugars the least.

Glycemic Load (GL): A true measure of the effect of a carbohydrate food on blood sugars based on two factors: the GI of that food and the amount consumed. GL=GI x amount of carbohydrate in the serve (in grams) divided by 100. Low GL= 0 -10; Medium GL= 10-20; High GL= >20. For example: 2 slices of multigrain bread contains 30g/1oz of carbohydrate.

Multigrain bread has a GI of 43. The GL of that serve= 43x30/100 = 13 and is considered a medium Glycemic Load.

Glycogen: A small reserve of stored sugar (glucose) found in the liver and muscle that the body can resort to, to prevent blood sugars from dropping too low—for example when a person burns up too much sugar during exercise or goes without food for extended periods of time (fasting).

Glycogenolysis: The process of converting stores of glycogen in the liver and muscle to sugar when blood sugars drop too low—for example during exercise or fasting. This process is carried out by a hormone called Glucagon produced in the pancreas.

High Density Lipoprotein cholesterol (HDL): Known as the good cholesterol. It carries excess cholesterol from cells to the liver and is a major factor protecting people from cardio-vascular disease.

Herbivore: An animal that lives on plant food alone. Examples include cows, sheep and goats.

Hormone: A chemical substance produced by an endocrine gland, whose secretions are delivered directly into the bloodstream and transported to a distant part or parts of the body, where they exert a specific effect for the benefit of the body as a whole. An example is the hormone insulin produced by the pancreas and affecting sugar uptake into muscle and fat cells.

Hydrogenation: A commercial process where refined liquid oils like soybean oil or canola oil are converted to hard fats like margarine and shortening by saturating carbon atoms in fatty acids with hydrogen at high temperatures of 120 to 210 degrees centigrade. This process is the most common way of drastically changing natural oils and causing the formation of bad 'trans fatty acids' in the process.

Hyperglycemia: High blood sugars—when if high enough—can result in one or more obvious symptoms like frequent urination, unusual thirst, excessive drinking, fatigue and blurred vision.

Hyperinsulinemia: A condition referring to abnormally high levels of insulin in the blood stream which can be caused by insulin resistance. These high levels of insulin are thought to result in diabetes, abnormal blood fats and increased cardiovascular disease.

Hypertension: A condition referring to abnormally high blood pressure.

Hypoglycemia: Lower than normal blood sugar levels- when if too low- can cause unusual symptoms of intense hunger, perspiration, light headedness, tiredness, confusion and the inability to concentrate. It occurs mostly in people treated with insulin injections, some blood sugar tablets but rarely if treated by diet and exercise alone.

Impaired Fasting Glucose (IFG): A pre-diabetic state where blood sugar levels after fasting overnight are higher than normal (5.6 to 6.9 mmol/l; 100 to 125 mg/dl) but not high enough to be classified as diabetic. This is associated with lower than normal levels of insulin being produced by the pancreas.

Impaired Glucose Tolerance (IGT): A pre-diabetic state that occurs when blood sugars two hours after meals are higher than normal (between 7.8 and 11 mmol/l; 140 to 198 mg/dl) but not high enough to be classified as diabetic. It is common in people with insulin resistance and central obesity.

Industrial Revolution: The period in human history when machines replaced manual labour in the second half of the 18th century. The revolution transformed agricultural economics into industrial ones causing far reaching social changes including movement of people from the land to cities.

Insulin: A hormone produced by the beta cells in the pancreas and secreted into the blood stream to help normalise blood sugar levels after meals. Insulin helps transfer glucose from the blood stream into muscle and fat cells where it is used as a source of fuel.

Insulin receptors: Are 'keyholes' on muscle and fat cells that insulin, like a 'key', normally binds to, to open doors allowing the transfer of sugar (glucose) from the blood stream into these cells. When this process does not work properly, insulin resistance and high blood sugars follow.

Insulin resistance (IR): A state when the hormone insulin, produced by the pancreas, is unable to do its job transferring sugars from the blood stream into muscle and fat cells. Glucose build-up in the blood stream can gradually follow resulting in Type 2 diabetes and increasing the risk of cardiovascular disease.

Joule: Is a unit of energy (heat) that is slowly replacing the calorie (see Calorie). A calorie is equal to 4.184 joules. One Calorie (capital C) = 1000 calories (small c) = one kilocalorie = 4.184 kilojoules (symbol kJ).

Ketoacidosis: A serious condition in Type 1 patients caused by high blood sugars and high levels of ketones in the blood stream. This is an emergency requiring hospitalisation.

Ketones: Are acidic substances produced by the body as alternative fuels to sugar (glucose) in people with Type 1 diabetes with very high blood sugars caused by inadequate insulin or illness. They are the result of fast breakdown of fat reserves and include acetone (nail polish!!), acetoacetate and betahydroxybutyrate that give their breath and urine a characteristic sweet acidic smell.

Lactase: Is the enzyme in the gut that helps digest or break down lactose into its components: glucose and galactose. Lactose intolerance can result if levels of lactase in the gut are lower than normal.

Lactose: A sugar that gives milk its sweet taste. It is a disaccharide made up of one molecule of glucose linked to one molecule of galactose. Lactose = glucose + galactose.

Lactose intolerance: The inability to digest lactose—the sugar in milk. Symptoms include flatus (gas), bloat and diarrhoea. It is treated by eliminating lactose from the diet i.e. using lactose—free dairy products.

Low Density Lipoprotein Cholesterol (LDL): Known as the bad cholesterol because high levels can block arteries and cause cardiovascular disease.

Linoleic acid (LA, 18:2 w6): An 18 carbon fatty acid of the omega 6 series with 2 double bonds. It is one of the two essential fatty acids. The body can not make it, requires it to stay healthy and must obtain it from food. Deficiency causes serious problems. LA rich foods include: the seeds and oils of safflower, sunflower, hemp and soybeans.

Linolenic acid (ALA): see alpha linolenic acid.

Lipids: The collective biochemical name for fats, oils, cholesterol and other fatty substances. Blood lipids refer to cholesterol and triglycerides in the blood.

Maltose: A sugar commonly known as malt. It is a disaccharide made up of one molecule of glucose linked up with another molecule of glucose. Maltose = glucose + glucose.

Metabolic Syndrome: A cluster of abnormalities associated with central (abdominal) obesity and insulin resistance and include high blood sugars, abnormal blood fats (high triglycerides and low HDL cholesterol) and high blood pressure among others.

Mg/dl: A measure of concentration in milligrams per decilitre or 100 millilitres of blood.

mm Hg: Millimetres of mercury—a measure of blood pressure. Although many modern vascular pressure devices no longer use mercury, blood pressure values are still universally reported in millimetres of mercury.

Mmol/l: A measure of concentration in millimoles per litre of blood.

Monosaccharide: A simple basic sugar. Examples include: Glucose, Fructose and Galactose.

Monounsaturated oil: Is made up largely of fatty acids containing only one double bond in their carbon chain. These are known to reduce cholesterol without affecting the good HDL cholesterol thus reducing the risk of cardiovascular disease. Olive oil and canola oil are good examples.

Negative energy balance: Is when energy output exceeds energy intake from food resulting in weight loss.

Nephropathy: A kidney disease that occurs as a result of poorly controlled diabetes. After many years of exposure to high blood sugars, the delicate filtering system in the kidney becomes destroyed, initially becoming leaky to large blood proteins such as albumin which are then lost in urine. It is a leading cause of kidney failure.

Normoglycemia: Normal blood glucose levels.

Omega 3 fats: A class of polyunsaturated fats essential to human health but lacking in the Western diet. We need to obtain more of these from our diet for normal growth, brain and eye development and prevention of cardiovascular disease. They are known to reduce triglycerides in the blood, reduce the stickiness of platelets and thin the blood preventing clot formation. For example: fish oils.

Omnivore: An animal that can live on both plant foods and animal flesh. For example: humans.

Oral Glucose Tolerance Test (OGTT): A laboratory test carried out to check ones sugar status. The person is asked to drink a solution containing 75 grams of sugar (glucose) after an overnight fast and their blood sugars are tested regularly over a two hour period. If blood sugar levels are less than 7.8 mmol/l two hours after the challenge they have normal glucose tolerance. If blood sugars are 7.8 to 11 they have Impaired Glucose Tolerance (IGT). If blood sugars are greater than 11.1 the person has diabetes.

Orlistat: A drug marketed under the name Xenical™ and designed to treat obesity. Its primary function is to prevent the absorption of fats from the diet thereby reducing energy intake.

Paleolithic Period: The Old Stone Age period of human evolution that began with Homo Habilis two million years ago and characterized by a hunter/gatherer way of life.

Peripheral neuropathy: Damage caused to nerves in the feet by exposure to high levels of blood sugars over time. It is a microvascular complication in people with badly controlled diabetes.

Peripheral vascular disease (PVD): Like other vascular diseases (heart disease and stroke), PVD is a disease of blocked arteries in the legs reducing the flow of blood to the lower extremities and increasing the risk of foot ulcers in people with diabetes.

Photosynthesis: The process by which plants make carbohydrate (sugar and starch) by combining water from the roots and carbon dioxide from the air with energy from the sun. Animals are unable to do so and thus rely on plants alone for their source of sugar.

Polycystic Ovary Syndrome (PCOS): A condition associated with insulin resistance and found in up to 5 to 10 per cent of females in their reproductive years. Symptoms include: irregular menstrual cycles, infertility, and male-like hormone secretions with excess face and body hair, male-like baldness, acne and oily skin. Treatment includes hormones, weight loss, regular activity and drugs to help improve insulin sensitivity.

Polyunsaturated Oils: Are made up largely of polyunsaturated fatty acids that contain at least one double bond in their carbon chain. These are known to reduce cholesterol and are found in liquid vegetable oils like sunflower, safflower and corn oils.

Postprandial glucose: Refers to blood sugar levels after meals (normally two hours in clinical practice).

Pre-diabetes: A stage where one has either Impaired Glucose Tolerance (IGT) or Impaired Fasting Glucose (IFG) that could progress to diabetes if lifestyle changes including weight loss, a proper diet and regular exercise are not practiced.

Processed: See 'refined'.

Reductil™: A drug used today to reduce appetite and help weight loss.

Refined: Refers to processed sugars, starches, fats and oils. Essential nutrients are removed from foods in the process robbing the body of their stores. In health terms 'refined' means 'processed' or 'deficient'.

Resistance exercise: Activity that consists of 'using muscle strength to move a weight or working against a resistance load'. Examples include weight lifting and exercise using weight machines.

Retinopathy: Damage to the retina of the eye caused by exposure to high blood sugars over time. It is a microvascular complication of people with badly controlled diabetes and a common cause of blindness.

Saturated fat: A fat made up largely of saturated fatty acids with no double bonds in the carbon chain. These are the bad fats that raise bad LDL cholesterol increasing the risk of cardiovascular disease. These are fats that are hard at room temperature like butter, suet and the fat off your beef or lamb chop.

Solvent extraction: The first step in the extraction of oil from seeds and nuts. Unlike in the case of mechanical pressing, this uses a chemical solvent such as hexane or heptane. Once the oil is extracted the solvent is then evaporated at a temperature of 150 degrees centigrade. Traces of these solvents may remain in the oil.

Starch: A carbohydrate made up of many glucose molecules (polysaccharide) linked together either in a branched (see Amylopectin) or in a straight chain (see Amylose) form. Examples include potato, rice, bread and pasta.

Statins: A class of drugs that stops the body making the bad LDL cholesterol. They include drugs like Atorvastatin (Lipitor™), Simvastatin (Lipex™), Pravastatin (Pravachol™), Rosuvastatin (Crestor™).

Subcutaneous fat: Fat deposited in the form of triglycerides underneath the skin all over the body when people gain weight. As opposed to abdominal or visceral fat, it is metabolised differently and has far less significance on health.

Sucrose: Commonly known as table sugar is a disaccharide made up of one molecule of glucose linked to one molecule of fructose. Sucrose = glucose + fructose.

Sulphonylureas: A group of drugs used to manage blood sugars in diabetes. They boost the pancreas to produce more insulin. Examples include Diamicron™, Diamicron MR™, Minidiab™ and Glimel™.

Systolic blood pressure: See Blood pressure.

Trans fatty acid (TFA): A type of unsaturated fatty acid where the hydrogen atoms on the carbons involved in a double bond are found on opposite sides of the molecule. It can impact on health by adversely raising the bad LDL cholesterol and reducing the good HDL cholesterol. It is found in small amounts in beef and lamb but is largely formed in the food manufacturing industry where vegetable oils are hydrogenated (processed) to act like animal fats.

Triglyceride: (TG): A basic molecule of animal fat or vegetable oil. It consists of three fatty acids linked to one molecule of glycerol. This is the form in which fatty acids are stored in the body's fatty tissues and in food (for example: meats, seeds and nuts). The body is capable of converting any surplus food that you eat (protein, fat, carbohydrate, or alcohol) into triglycerides and storing it away for a rainy day. A great survival mechanism!

Urbanisation: The movement of people from the land to the city and its lifestyle changes.

This often corresponds to a significant increase in diabetes.

Visceral fat: Fat stored in the form of triglycerides deep in the abdominal or waistline area. This fat is thought to be metabolised differently to fat stored underneath the skin (subcutaneous). Unlike subcutaneous fat, it increases insulin resistance, the risk of diabetes and cardiovascular complications.

Vitamin E: An essential vitamin needed by the body and found in nut and seed oils where it acts as a natural antioxidant to protect the oil from spoiling.

Xenical™: See Orlistat.

REFERENCES

1. Eaton SB, et al. 2002. Evolutionary health promotion. Preventive Medicine 34: 109-118.

2. Eaton SB, Konner M. 1985. Paleolithic nutrition: a consideration of its nature and current implications. New Engl J Med 312: 283-289.

3. American Diabetes Association. 2000. Type 2 diabetes in children and adolescents. Diabetes Care 23: 381-389.

4. Fagot-Campana A, et al. 2000. Type 2 diabetes among North American children and adolescents: an epidemiological review and a public health perspective. J Pediatrics 136: 664-672.

5. Laurencin MG, et al. 2005. Type 2 diabetes in adolescents. How to recognize and treat this growing problem. (Review). Post-graduate Medicine 118 (5): 31-36, 43.

6. Eppens MC, et al. 2006. Prevalence of diabetes complications in adolescents with Type 2 compared with Type 1 diabetes. Diabetes Care 29 (6): 1300-1306.

7. Reaven GM. 1995. Pathophysiology of insulin resistance in human disease. Physiol. Rev. 75: 473-486.

8. Sicree R, et al. 2003. The Global Burden of diabetes. In: Gan D, ed. Diabetes Atlas. 2nd ed. Brussels, Belgium: International Diabetes Federatio: 15-71.

9. Dunstan DW, et al. 2002. The rising prevalence of diabetes and impaired glucose tolerance: the Australian Diabetes, Obesity and Lifestyle Study. Diabetes Care 25 (5): 829-834.

10. Barr E, et al 2006. 'AusDiab 2005. The Australian Diabetes, Obesity and Lifestyle Study', International Diabetes Institute, Melbourne.

11. Australian Institute of Health and Welfare. 2008. Diabetes: Australian facts 2008. Diabetes series no. 8. Cat. No. CVD 40. Canberra: AIHW.

12. Mokdad AH, et al. 2000. Diabetes Trends in the U.S.: 1990-1998. Diabetes Care 23 (9): 1278-128.

13. Mokdad AH, et al. 2001. The continuing Epidemics of Obesity and Diabetes in the United States. J Am Med Assoc 286: 1195-1200.

14. Mokdad AH, et al. 2003. Prevalence of Obesity, Diabetes, and Obesity- Related Health Risk Factors, 2001. JAMA 289 (1): 76-79.

15. Schulz LO, et al. 2006. Effects of traditional and Western environments on prevalence of type 2 diabetes in Pima Indians in Mexico and the US. Diabetes Care 29: 1866-1871.

16. Colditz GA, et al. 1990. Weight as a risk factor for clinical diabetes in women. Am J Epidemiol 132: 501-513.

17. Zimmet P, 2007. Diabesity- The biggest Epidemic in Human History. Medscape General Medicine 9 (3): 39.

18. Pouliot MC, et al. 1994. Waist circumference and abdominal sagittal diameter: best simple anthropometric indexes of ab-dominal visceral adipose tissue accumulation and related cardiovascular risk in men and women. Am J Cardiol 73: 460-468.

19. Carey VJ, et al. 1997. Body fat distribution and risk of non-insulin dependant diabetes mellitus in women: the Nurses' Health Study. Am J Epidemiol 145: 614-619.

20. Nestle M. 2006. Food marketing and childhood obesity – a matter of policy. N Engl J Med. 354: 2527-2529.

21. Cameron AJ, et al. 2003. Overweight and obesity in Australia: the 1999-2000 Australian diabetes, Obesity and Lifestyle Study (Ausdiab). Medical Journal of Australia 178: 427-432.

22. Pan XR, et al. 1997. Effects of diet and exercise in preventing NIDDM in people with impaired glucose tolerance. The DaQ-ing IGT and Diabetes Study. Diabertes Care 20: 537-544.

23. Tuomilehto J, et al. 2001. Prevention of type 2 diabetes mellitus by changes in lifestyle among subjects with impaired glu-cose tolerance. New Eng J Med 344: 1343-1350.

24. Knowler WC, et al. 2002. Reduction in the incidence of Type 2 diabetes with lifestyle intervention or metformin. New Eng J Med 346: 393-403.

25. Laakso M, 2005. Prevention of Type 2 diabetes. Current Molecular Medicine 5 (3): 365-374.

26. Ramachandran A, et al. 2006. The Indian Diabetes Prevention Programme shows that lifestyle modification and metformin prevent type 2 diabetes in Asian Indian subjects with impaired glucose tolerance (IDDP-1). Diabetologia 49: 289-297.

27. Chiasson JL, et al 2002. Acarbose for the prevention of Type 2 diabetes mellitus: the STOP-NIDDM randomised trial. Lancet 359: 2072-2077.

28. The DREAM trial investigators. 2006. Effect of rosiglitazone on the frequency of diabetes in patients with impaired glucose tolerance or impaired fasting glucose: a randomised controlled trial. The Lancet 368: 1096-1105.

29. Gabir MG, et al. 2000. The 1997 American Diabetes Association and 1999 World Health Organization criteria for hyperglycemia in the diagnosis and prediction of diabetes. Diabetes Care 23: 1108-1112.

30. Borch-Johnsen K, et al.2004. Creating a pandemic of prediabetes: the proposed new diagnostic criteria for impaired fasting glycaemia. Diabetologia 47: 1396-1402.

31. Peterson JL, McGuire DK. 2005. Impaired glucose tolerance and impaired fasting glucose—a review of diagnosis, clinical implications and management. (Review). Diabetes & Vascular Disease Research 2 (1): 9-15.

32. O'Keefe JH, Cordain L. 2004. Cardiovascular disease resulting from a diet and lifestyle at odds with our Paleolithic Genome: How to become a 21st century Hunter-Gatherer. Mayo Clin Proceedings 79: 101-108.

33. Cordain L, et al. 2006a. Origins and evolution of the Western diet: health implications for the 21st century. American Journal of Clinical Nutrition 81 (2): 341-354.

34. Cordain L, et al. 2006b. Plant-animal subsistence ratios and macronutrient energy estimations in worldwide hunter-gatherer diets. American Journal of Clinical Nutrition 71 (3): 682-692.

35. O'Dea K. 1984. Marked improvement in carbohydrate and lipid metabolism in diabetic Australian Aborigines after temporary reversion to traditional lifestyle. Diabetes 33(6): 596-603.

36. Eckel, RH et al. 2005. The metabolic syndrome. The Lancet 365: 1415-1428.

37. Gami AS, et al. 2007. Metabolic syndrome and risk of incident cardiovascular events and death: a systematic review and meta-analysis of longitudinal studies. J Am Coll Cardiol. 49: 403-414.

38. Grundy SM, et al. 2005a. Diagnosis and management of the metabolic syndrome. An American Heart Association /National Heart, Lung, and Blood Institute Scientific Statement. Circulation 112: 2735-2752.

39. Alberti G, et al. 2005. The metabolic syndrome—a new worldwide definition for the IDF epidemiology task force consensus group. The Lancet 366: 1059-1062.

40. Despres JP, Lemieux,I. 2006. Abdominal obesity and metabolic syndrome. Nature 444 (7121): 881-887.

41. Zimmet P, et al. 2007. The metabolic syndrome in children and adolescents- an IDF consensus report. Pediatric Diabetes 8: 299–306.

42. Alexander CM, et al. 2003. Third National Health and Nutrition Examination Survey (NHANES III); National Cholesterol Education Program (NCEP). NCEP-defined metabolic syndrome, diabetes, and prevalence of coronary heart disease among NHANES III participants age 50 years and older. Diabetes. 52 (5): 1210-1214.

43. International Diabetes Federation. 2003. Diabetes Atlas, Second Edition.

44. Wyne Kl. 2005. Metabolic Syndrome: demographic features, etiology and clinical management. (Review). Current Atherosclerosis Report. 7 (5): 381-388.

45. International Diabetes Federation 2007. Guidelines for management of postmeal glucose. www.idf.org

46. The Diabetes Control and Complications Trial Research Group.1993. The effect of intensive treatment of diabetes on the development and progression of long-term complications in insulin—dependent diabetes mellitus. New Eng J Med 329: 977-986.

47. The Diabetes Control and Complications Trial/Epidemiology of Diabetes Interventions and Complications (DCCT/EDIC) Study Research Group. 2005. Intensive Diabetes Treatment and Cardiovascular Disease in Patients with Type 1 Diabetes. New Eng J Med 353: 2643-2653.

48. Coutinho M, et al. 1999. The relationship between glucose and incident cardiovascular events. A metaregression analysis of published data from 20 studies of 95,783 individuals followed for 12.4 years. Diabetes Care 22 (2): 233-240.

49. Harrison's Principles of Internal Medicine. 2005. 16th Edition. The McGraw—Hills Companies, Inc. Kasper DL et al Editors.

50. Best J, et al. 2004. Evidence based guidelines for Type 2 Diabetes: Lipid control. Diabetes Australia & NHMRC, Canberra.

51. Resnick HE, et al. 2000. American Diabetes Association diabetes diagnostic criteria, advancing age, and cardiovascular disease risk profiles: results from the Third National Health and Nutrition Examination Survey. Diabetes Care 23: 176-180.

52. Kannel WB. 1983. High-density lipoproteins: epidemiologic profile and risks of coronary artery disease. Am J Cardiol. 52: 9B-12B.

53. Castelli WP. 1992. Epidemiology of triglycerides: a view from Framingham. Am J Cardiol. 70: 3H-9H.

54. Sarwar N, et al. 2007. Triglycerides and the risk of coronary heart disease: 10,158 incident cases among 262,525 participants in 29 Western prospective studies. Circulation. 115(4): 450-458.

55. Garvey WT, et al. 2003. Effects of insulin resistance and type 2 diabetes on lipoprotein subclass particle size and concentration determined by nuclear magnetic resonance. Diabetes. 52(2): 453-462.

56. Brohall G, et al. 2006. Carotid artery intima-media thickness in patients with Type 2 diabetes mellitus and impaired glucose tolerance: a systematic review. Diabet Med 23(6): 609-616.

57. Newman H, et al. 2004. Evidence based guidelines for Type 2 Diabetes: Macrovascular disease. Diabetes Australia & NHMRC, Canberra.

58. Cholesterol Treatment Trialists' (CTT) Collaborators. 2005. Efficacy and safety of cholesterol-lowering treatment: prospective meta-analysis of data from 90,056 participants in 14 randomised trials of statins. Lancet. 366: 1267-1278.

59. Scandinavian Simvastatin Survival Study (4S) Group. 1994. Randomised trial of cholesterol lowering in 4444 patients with coronary heart disease: the Scandinavian Simvastatin Survival Study (4S). Lancet 344: 1383-1389.

60. Downs JR, et al. 1998. Primary prevention of acute coronary events with Lovastatin in men and women with average cholesterol levels: results of the AFCAPS/TexCAPS. Air Force/Texas Coronary Atherosclerosis Prevention Study. JAMA 279: 1615-1622.

61. Sacks FM, et al. 1998. Relationship between plasma LDL concentrations during treatment with pravastatin and recurrent coronary events in the Cholesterol and Recurrent Events Trial. Circulation 97: 1446-1452.

62. Costa J, et al. 2006. Efficacy of lipid lowering drug treatment for diabetic and non-diabetic patients: meta-analysis of randomised controlled trials. BMJ 332: 1115-1124.

63. Shepherd J, et al. 2006. Effect of lowering LDL cholesterol substantially below currently recommended levels in patients with coronary heart disease and diabetes: the Treating to New Targets (TNT) study. Diabetes Care 29: 1220-1226.

64. Manninen V, et al. 1992. Joint effects of serum triglyceride and LDL cholesterol and HDL cholesterol concentrations on coronary heart disease risk in the Helsinki Heart Study: implications for treatment. Circulation 85: 37-45.

65. Rubins HB, et al. for the VA-HIT Study Group. 2002. Diabetes, plasma insulin, and cardiovascular disease: subgroup analysis from the Department of Veterans Affairs high-density lipoprotein intervention trial (VA-HIT). Arch Intern Med .162: 2597-2604.

66. Keech A, et al. 2005. Effects of long-term fenofibrate therapy on cardiovascular events in 9795 people with type 2 diabetes mellitus (the FIELD study): randomised controlled trial. The Lancet 366: 1849-1861.

67. Durrington PN, et al. 2001. An omega-3 polyunsaturated fatty acid concentrate administered for one year decreased triglycerides in simvastatin treated patients with coronary heart disease and persisting hypertriglyceridaemia. Heart 85: 544-548.

68. Grundy SM, et al. 2005b. Effectiveness and tolerability of simvastatin plus fenofibrate for combined hyperlipidemia (the SAFARI trial). Am J Cardiol 95: 462-468.

69. Brown BG, et al. 2001. Simvastatin and niacin, antioxidant vitamins, or the combination for the prevention of coronary disease. N Engl J Med. 345: 1583-1592.

70. Arner P, 1997. Regional adiposity in man. J Endocrinology 155: 191-192.

71. Klein S, et al. 2004. Weight management through lifestyle modification for the prevention and management of Type 2 diabetes: Rationale and strategies. A statement of the American Diabetes Association, the North American Association for the Study of Obesity, and the American Society for Clinical Nutrition. Diabetes Care 27: 2067-2073.

72. Cummings DE, Flum DR. 2008. Gastrointestinal surgery as a treatment for diabetes. JAMA 299 (3): 341-343.

73. Goodpaster BH, et al 2005. Obesity, regional body fat distribution, and the metabolic syndrome in older women. Arch Intern Med 165: 777-783.

74. Piche M, et al. 2005. Contribution of abdominal visceral obesity and insulin resistance to the cardiovascular risk profile of postmenopausal women. Diabetes 54: 770-777.

75. Fried SK, et al. 1998. Omental and subcutaneous adipose tissues of obese subjects release interleukin-6: depot difference and regulation by glucocorticoid. J Clin Endocrinol Metab 83: 847-850.

76. Gomi T, et al. 2005. Measurement of Visceral Fat/subcutaneous Fat Ratio by 0.3 Tesla MRI. Radiation Medicine 23 (8): 584-587.

77. Atkins RC. 1998. Dr Atkins' The New Diet Revolution. New York, NY: Avon Books.

78. Pedrini MT, et al. 1996. The effect of dietary protein restriction on the progression of diabetic and non-diabetic renal diseases: a meta-analysis. Ann Inter Med 124: 627-632.

79. Pijls LT, et al. 1999. The effect of protein restriction on albuminuria in patients with type 2 diabetes mellitus: a randomized trial. Nephrol Dial Transplant 14: 1445-1453.

80. Hansen HP, et al. 2002. Effect of dietary protein restriction on prognosis in patients with diabetic nephropathy. Kidney Int 62: 220-228.

81. Ornish D. 1990. Dr. Dean Ornish's Program for Reversing Heart Disease: The Only System Scientifically Proven to reverse Heart Disease without Drugs or Surgery. New York, NY. Random House.

82. Brinkworth GD, et al. 2004. Long-term effects of advice to consume high -protein , low-fat diet, rather than a conventional weight-loss diet, in obese adults with Type 2 diabetes: one-year follow-up of a randomised trial. Diabetologia 47 (10): 1677 to 1686.

83. Noakes M, Clifton P. 2004. Weight loss, diet composition and cardiovascular risk. Current Opinion in Lipidology 15: 31-35.

84. Noakes M, Clifton P. 2005. The CSIRO total wellbeing diet. Penguin Group (Australia).

85. Jerums G, et al. 2004. Evidence based guidelines for Type 2 Diabetes: Blood Pressure control. Diabetes Australia & NHMRC, Canberra.

86. American Diabetes Association. 2004a. Nutrition principles and recommendations in diabetes. Diabetes Care 27 (suppl 1): S36-S46.

87. American Diabetes Association. 2004b. Physical activity/Exercise and diabetes. Diabetes Care 27 (suppl 1): S58-S62.

88. Thomas DE, et al. 2006. Exercise for type 2 diabetes mellitus. Cochrane Database of Systematic Reviews, Issue 3. Art No. CD002968

89. Atlantis E, et al. 2007. Weight status and perception barriers to healthy physical activity and diet behaviour. International Journal of Obesity advance online publication, 7 August.

90. Medibank Private. 2007. The cost of physical inactivity. What is the lack of participation in physical activity costing Australia?

91. Booth FW, et al. 2000. Waging war on modern chronic diseases: primary prevention through exercise biology. J Appl Physiol 88: 774-787.

92. McGinnis JM, Foege WH. 1993. Actual causes of death in the United States. JAMA: 270: 2207-2212.

93. Cordain L, et al. 1998. Physical activity, energy expenditure and fitness: an evolutionary perspective. International Journal of Sports Medicine 19: 328-335.

94. Laaksonen DE, et al. 2005. Physical activity in the prevention of Type 2 diabetes: the Finnish Diabetes Prevention Study. Diabetes 54 (1): 158-165.

95. Ivy JL. 1997. Role of exercise training in the treatment of insulin resistance and non-insulin-dependant diabetes mellitus. Sports Med 24: 321-336.

96. Boule NG, et al. 2001. Effects of exercise on glycemic control and body mass in Type 2 diabetes mellitus: a meta-analysis of controlled clinical trials. JAMA 286: 1218-1227.

97. Thomas N, et al. 2004. Barriers to physical activity in patients with diabetes. Postgrad Med J 80: 287-291.

98. Catenacci VA, Wyatt HR. 2007. The role of physical activity in producing and maintaining weight loss. Nat Clin Pract Endocrinol Metab 3 (7): 518-529.

99. Wing RR. 1999. Physical activity in the treatment of adulthood overweight and obesity: current evidence and research issues. Med Sci Sports Exerc. 31 (11, suppl): S547-S552.

100. Albright A, et al. 2000. American College of Sports Medicine position stand: exercise and type 2 diabetes. Med Sci Sports Exerc 32: 1345-1360.

101. Boule NG, et al 2003. Meta-analysis of the effect of structured exercise training on cardiovascular respiratory fitness in type 2 diabetes mellitus. Diabetologia 46: 1071-1081.

102. NHMRC publications. 2005. Nutrient Reference Values for Australia and New Zealand. Including Recommended Dietary Intakes. www.nhmrc.gov.au/publications

103. Malouf N, Colagiuri R, Colagiuri S. 1993. Evaluation of a new healthy food pyramid for diabetes. Proceedings of the Australian Diabetes Educators Association Annual meeting, Abstract E8.

104. Malouf N, Turner L, Colagiuri S. 2004. A 'Diet Kit' for diabetes educators. ADS & ADEA Annual Scientific Meeting Proceedings and abstracts. Abstract pp 178.

105. The Traffic Light Guide to Food. 2005 Ed. The Diabetes Education Centre- Royal North Shore Hospital, St Leonards, Sydney NSW, Australia 2065.

106. Ello-Martin JA, et al. 2007. Dietary energy density in the treatment of obesity: a year-long trial comparing two weight-loss diets. Am J Clin Nutr 85:1465-1477.

107. NHMRC publications. 2003. Dietary Guidelines for Australian Adults. www.nhmrc.gov.au/publications

108. Sheard NF, et al. 2004. Dietary carbohydrate (amount and type) in the prevention and management of diabetes: a statement by the American Diabetes Association. (Reviews/Commentaries/ADA Statements). Diabetes Care 27: 2266-2271.

109. Wolever TMS, et al. 2006. Food glycemic index, as given in Glycemic Index tables, is a significant determinant of glycemic responses elicited by composite breakfast meals. Am J Clin Nutr 83 (6): 1306-1312.

110. Jenkins DJ, et al.1981. Glycemic index of foods: a physiological basis for carbohydrate exchange. Am J Clin Nutr 34: 362-366.

111. Miller JB, et al. 1998. The GI factor. The Gycaemic Index solution. Second edition. Published by Hodder Headline Australia Pty Ltd.

112. Miller JB, et al. 2003. The New Glucose Revolution. 3rd edition. Published by Hodder Headline Australia Pty Ltd.

113. Thorburn AW, et al. 1987. Slowly digested and absorbed carbohydrate in traditional bushfoods: a protective factor against diabetes? Am J Clin Nutr. 45: 98-106.

114. Australian Bureau of Statistics: Commonwealth Department of Health and Aged Care. 1998. National Nutrition Survey. Nutrient intakes and physical measurements, Australia 1995. Canberra: Australian Bureau of Statistics.

115. Cordain L, et al. 2002. Fatty acid analysis of wild ruminant tissues: evolutionary implications for reducing diet-related chronic disease. Eur J Clin Nutr 56: 181-191.

116. Sinclair AJ, et al. 1998. The omega-3 fatty acid content of canned, smoked and fresh fish in Australia. Aust J Nutr Diet 55: 116-120.

117. Mori TA. 1999. Fish oils, dyslipidaemia and glycaemic control in diabetes. Pract Diabetes Int 16: 223-226.

118. Gylling H, Miettinen TA. 1999. Cholesterol reduction by different plant stanol mixtures and with variable fat intake. Metabolism 48: 575-580.

119. Hu FB, et al. 1998. Frequent nut consumption and risk of coronary heart disease in women: prospective cohort study. BMJ 317: 1341-1345.

120. Fraser GE, Shavlik DJ. 1997. Risk factors for all-cause and coronary heart disease mortality in the oldest-old. The Adventist Health Study. Arch Intern Med 157: 2249-2258.

121. Garg A. 1998. High mono-unsaturated fat diets for patients with diabetes mellitus: a meta-analysis. Am J Clin Nutrition 67 (Suppl 1): 577-582.

122. Hulthe J, Fagerberg B. 2005. Alcohol consumption and insulin sensitivity: A review. Metabol Synd Rel Disord 3: 45-50.

123. Beulens J, et al. 2005. Alcohol consumption and risk of type 2 diabetes among older women. Diabetes Care 28: 2933-2938.

124. Koppes LLJ, et al. 2005. Moderate alcohol consumption lowers the risk of Type 2 diabetes. Diabetes Care 28 (3): 719-725.

125. Fan A, et al. 2006. Lifetime alcohol drinking pattern is related to the prevalence of metabolic syndrome. The Western New York Health Study (WNYHS). Eur J Epidemiol 21: 129 -138.

126. Wei M, et al.2000. Alcohol intake and incidence of type 2 diabetes in men. Diabetes Care 23(1): 18–22.

127. Suter P. 2005. Is alcohol consumption a risk factor for weight gain and obesity? Crit Rev Clin Lab Sci 42: 197-227.

128. Foster R, Marriott H. 2006. Alcohol consumption in the new millennium—weighing up the risks and benefits for our health. Nutr Bull 31: 286-331.

129. Arif AA, Rohrer JE. 2005. Patterns of alcohol drinking and its association with obesity: Data from the third national health and nutrition examination survey, 1988–1994. BMC Pub Health 5: 126.

130. Howard AA, et al. 2004. Effect of alcohol consumption on Diabetes Mellitus. A systematic review. Ann Intern Med 140: 211-219.

131. Cheyne E, et al. 2004. Influence of alcohol on cognitive performance during mild hypoglycaemia; implications for Type 1 diabetes. Diabet Med 21: 230-237.

ADDITIONAL RESOURCES

United Kingdom

Association for the study of obesity www.aso.org.uk

British Heart Foundation www.bhf.org.uk

British Nutrition Foundation www.nutrition.org.uk

Diabetes UK www.diabetes.org.uk

Heart UK www.heartuk.org.uk

United States

American Association of Diabetes Educators www.diabeteseducator.org

American Diabetes Association www.diabetes.org

American Dietetic Association www.eatright.org

American Heart Association www.americanheart.org

American Podiatric Medical Association www.apma.org

Centers for Disease Control (CDC) Atlanta, USA www.cdc.gov/diabetes

Joslin Diabetes centre www.joslin.org

Juvenile Diabetes Foundation (JDF) www.jdrf.org

International organisations

International Association for the Study of Obesity IASO www.iaso.org

International Diabetes Federation—Global perspectives on diabetes www.diabetesvoice.org , www.idf.org

Australia

Australian Association for Exercise and Sport Science (AAESS) www.aaess.com.au

Australian Diabetes Educators Association www.adea.com.au

Australian Heart Foundation www.heartfoundation.com.au

Australian Podiatry Council www.apodc.com.au

Calorie, Fat & Carbohydrate counter www.CalorieKing.com.au

Diabetes Australia www.diabetesaustralia.com.au

Diabetes Counselling Online www.diabetescounselling.com.au

Dietitians Association of Australia www.daa.asn.au

Glycemic Index www.glycemicindex.com

Glycemic Index Symbol www.gisymbol.com

International Diabetes Institute www.diabetes.com.au

Juvenile Diabetes Research Foundation www.jdrf.org.au

Lifestyle Clinic, University of New South Wales www.lifestyle-clinic.net.au

Nutrition Australia www.nutritionaustralia.org

Quitline. To help you stop smoking Tel: 131 848

The Australian dietary guidelines and Food for Health information can be found at www.nhmrc.gov.au/publications/nhome.htm

New Zealand

Diabetes New Zealand www.diabetes.org.nz

National Heart Foundation of New Zealand www.nhf.org.nz

New Zealand Dietetics Association www.dietitians.org.nz

New Zealand Register of Exercise Professionals www.reps.org.nz

New Zealand Society of Podiatrists www.podiatry.org.nz

Quitline. To help you stop smoking Tel: 0800778778

First published in Australia in 2009 by
New Holland Publishers (Australia) Pty Ltd
Sydney • Auckland • London • Cape Town

1/66 Gibbes Street Chatswood NSW 2067 Australia
218 Lake Road Northcote Auckland New Zealand
86 Edgware Road London W2 2EA United Kingdom
80 McKenzie Street Cape Town 8001 South Africa

A record of this book is held at the National Library of Australia

ISBN 9781741107616

Publisher: Fiona Schultz
Publishing Manager: Lliane Clarke
Editor: Kay Proos
Proofreader: Caroline Beaumont
Designer: Tania Gomes
Production Assistant: Liz Malcolm
Printer: SNP/Leefung Printing Co. Ltd (China)